Trauma in the Creative and Embodied Therapies

Trauma in the Creative and Embodied Therapies is a cross-professional book looking at current approaches to working therapeutically and socially with trauma in a creative and embodied way.

The book pays attention to different kinds of trauma – environmental, sociopolitical, early relational, abuse in its many forms, and the trauma of illness – with contributions from international experts, drawn from the fields of the arts therapies, the embodied psychotherapies, as well as nature-based therapy and Playback Theatre. The book is divided into three sections: the first section takes into consideration the wider sociopolitical perspective of trauma and the power of community engagement. In the second section, there are numerous clinical approaches to working with trauma, whether with individuals or groups, highlighting the importance of creative and embodied approaches. In the third section, the focus shifts from client work to the impact of trauma on the practitioner, team, and supervisor, and the importance of creative self-care and reflection in managing this challenging field.

This book will be useful for all those working in the field of trauma, whether as clinicians, artists, or social workers.

Anna Chesner is co-director of the London Centre for Psychodrama Group and Individual Psychotherapy, where she trains psychotherapists and supervisors. Anna works in private practice in London as a UKCP registered psychotherapist and supervisor.

sissy lykou, MA, PGCert, Onassis Foundation fellow, is a UKCP registered psychotherapist, dance movement psychotherapist and supervisor, and the programme leader of the MSc in Contemporary Person-Centred Psychotherapy at Metanoia Institute. She practises in London privately and in community psychotherapy projects for children under five years of age and their parents/carers. She is also the clinical community and outreach lead of an innovative therapists' community, Stillpoint Spaces London.

Trauma in the Creative and Embodied Therapies

When Words Are Not Enough

Edited by
Anna Chesner and sissy lykou

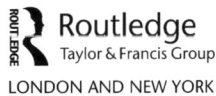

Routledge
Taylor & Francis Group

LONDON AND NEW YORK

First published 2021
by Routledge
2 Park Square, Milton Park, Abingdon, Oxon OX14 4RN

and by Routledge
52 Vanderbilt Avenue, New York, NY 10017

Routledge is an imprint of the Taylor & Francis Group, an informa business

British Library Cataloguing-in-Publication Data
A catalogue record for this book is available from the British Library

Library of Congress Cataloging-in-Publication Data
Names: Chesner, Anna, editor. | lykou, sissy, editor.
Title: Trauma in the creative and embodied therapies : when words are not enough / edited by Anna Chesner and sissy lykou.
Description: Abingdon, Oxon ; New York, NY : Routledge, 2021. |
Includes bibliographical references and index.
Identifiers: LCCN 2020014249 (print) | LCCN 2020014250 (ebook) |
ISBN 9781138479227 (hardback) | ISBN 9781138479210 (paperback) |
ISBN 9781351066266 (ebook)
Subjects: LCSH: Psychic trauma--Treatment. | Art therapy. |
Arts--Therapeutic use. | Drama--Therapeutic use. |
Mind and body therapies.
Classification: LCC RC552.T7 T7365 2020 (print) |
LCC RC552.T7 (ebook) |
DDC 616.89/1656--dc23
LC record available at https://lccn.loc.gov/2020014249
LC ebook record available at https://lccn.loc.gov/2020014250

ISBN: 9781138479227 (hbk)
ISBN: 9781138479210 (pbk)
ISBN: 9781351066266 (ebk)

Typeset in Sabon
by Taylor & Francis Books

To Yiorgos and Agelos

Contents

Figures

Foreword

This is a genuinely ground-breaking book on many fronts. It propels discussion about therapeutic approaches to trauma into new interdisciplinary territory. In this creative editorial partnership, Chesner and Iykou have assembled a very current and engaging set of contributions to the rapidly developing field of trauma therapies.

Freud's original conception of trauma, revolutionary in its time, has over decades expanded to include developmental trauma, PTSD, and intergenerational trauma. This book pays due attention to these types of trauma, and extends this into contemporary considerations. This includes sociopolitical and environmental trauma, highlighting the intersection between collective processes and individual trauma. A number of chapters explore multiple facets of early relational trauma, domestic and sexual violence, and other hidden traumas, such as the impact of medical procedures. An international set of authors reflect on their experience of working with diverse individuals and groups from around the world.

Even more striking is the boldness and breadth of therapies represented here: art, drama, dance movement and music therapies; play therapy; Gestalt, psychodrama psychotherapy, and body psychotherapy; integrative arts therapy and nature-based trauma therapy. I am delighted to see the inclusion of a chapter on Playback Theatre – a non-scripted, spontaneous drama medium rooted in storytelling used therapeutically in community settings. Its author, Jo Salas, quotes Bessel van der Kolk: "Without imagination there is no hope, no chance to envisage a better future, no place to go, no goal to reach." (2015, p. 17).

Reading this book really nourished my sense of the aliveness and healing potential of working in an embodied creative way. This is important because we are living in times in which multiple traumatising factors are converging on many children and adults, and health services are under great strain. Psychotherapists are having to find deeper resources within themselves to maintain generative, grounded, and sensitively attuned work with their clients. So it is appropriate and affirming that there are chapters on supervision and on therapists' experience of illness and recovery.

Trauma in the Creative and Embodied Therapies weaves together theory and clinical experience, demonstrating how science, art, inquiry, imagination, embodied exploration, and deep care are all part of the therapeutic journey "[W]hen words are not enough ..." The authors show they can focus on non-verbal affective implicit communication in the therapeutic relationship and utilise body-and-arts-based enactive means of unfolding stories, meanings, and healing relationships. The balance and interplay between group and individual work is well represented. The groupwork approaches – psychodrama psychotherapy, dance movement psychotherapy, and Turner's Model of Crisis – all draw in part on non-Western and indigenous traditions of healing.

The metaphor of a journey is often used to describe therapeutic work. And indeed therapeutic work does involve precisely the process of *moving through* stages of often excruciating, testing, heart-breaking, and chaotic relational and emotional landscapes. One step, fall, sound, twist, sentence, gather and reach at a time. These chapters are rich in moving and vivid case material with children and adults, individuals, and groups – the 'lost year' of Celeste, the psychic bomb inside Jerry, Nik's slide into the mud, and the story of a shared rice ball in a community of survivors of Fukushima.

What contains and supports psychotherapists, whether they are seasoned clinicians or trainees, is a sound and broad theoretical framework. These chapters cover a wide and contemporary range of trauma-informed, research-based psychotherapeutic thinking, from neuroscience, attachment theory, movement observation, auto-ethnographic, and feminist theories, as well as the unique meta-theories employed by the different arts-based approaches.

It is a book that will inspire and satisfy, educate and engage, expand and focus the attention of its readers on the healing potential of embodied creativity in trauma therapy.

Roz Carroll

Acknowledgements

We wish to thank our editor, Joanne Forshaw, for her warmth, kindness, and consistent availability. Her approach and guidance made this project a joy and a great learning process.

Anna

Anna would like to thank sissy for the co-working experience and give a particular thanks to the clients and trainees who contribute so much to the ongoing learning about trauma and clinical practice.

sissy

sissy owes a great deal to her family in Athens and their consistently open hug: Stavroula Lykou, Yiorgos Lykos, Maria Lykou, Kostas Marinidis, Michalis Sourmelakis, and little Yiorgos and Aggelos. This adventure would not have been fulfilled without her family in London too: Paul Christelis, Pieter Maritz, Aaron Balick, Begum Maitra, and Mónica Malfitano; their verbal and non-verbal motivation have been poignant. Special thanks to sissy's fellow-thinking travellers and comrades Ioanna Kousteni and Marina Rova for their ongoing support and encouragement. sissy wishes to acknowledge the influence in her work of two dear colleagues and friends who have been models for her for many years now: Suzanne Keys and Roz Carroll. sissy feels indebted to her clients who have trusted her and have allowed the unfolding of her ideas in the relationships with her. Finally, big, big thanks to her co-editor, Anna Chesner, for her trust and vision for this project and for her wise guidance in her baby-steps in editing.

Contributors

Anna Chesner, MA, UKCP registered psychotherapist and training supervisor is co-director of the London Centre for Psychodrama Group and Individual Psychotherapy. She is trained as a psychodrama psychotherapist, group analytic psychotherapist, dramatherapist, and Playback Theatre practitioner. She works as a psychotherapist and supervisor in private practice in London, and as a trainer in UK, Switzerland, and Hong Kong. She is widely published in the fields of psychodrama, dramatherapy, groupwork, and creative supervision.

sissy lykou, MA, PGCert, Onassis Foundation fellow, is a UKCP registered psychotherapist, dance movement psychotherapist and supervisor, and the programme leader of the MSc in Contemporary Person-Centred Psychotherapy at Metanoia Institute. She practises in London privately and in community psychotherapy projects for children under five years of age and their parents/carers. She lectures on several university and professional training programmes in the UK and Europe and has worked on EU research projects at the Universities of Heidelberg and Athens. In addition to publishing papers and chapters, she serves on journal editorial boards and was a member of the Steering Group of Psychotherapists and Counsellors for Social Responsibility. She has been the clinical community and outreach lead of Stillpoint Spaces London since its beginning: www.lykou counselling.co.uk.

Roz Carroll is a Chiron-trained relational body psychotherapist. She teaches "Contemporary Theories of Psychotherapy" on the MA in Integrative Psychotherapy at The Minster Centre and is a regular speaker for Confer. She is the author of numerous articles and chapters, including: "The Blood-dimmed Tide: Witnessing War and Working with the Collective Body in Authentic Movement" in the *Journal of Psychotherapy and Politics International* and "Four Relational Modes of Attending to the Body in Psychotherapy" in Ed. (2014) K. White *Talking Bodies: How do we Integrate Working with the Body in Psychotherapy from an Attachment and Relational Perspective?*

Sophia Condaris is an integrative arts psychotherapist (UKCP) and a dramatherapist (HCPC). She is presently the course leader for the dramatherapy masters programme at Anglia Ruskin University. Currently her clinical role is working with children and their families in the NHS. She has previously worked intensively with children who have a history of trauma and has close links with South Africa where she has run projects in communities affected by poverty and violence. She is also trainer at the Institute for Arts in Therapy and Education.

Dr Ditty Dokter is a registered dramatherapist (HCPC), dance movement psychotherapist (ADMP), and group analytic psychotherapist (UKCP). Her last clinical post was as professional lead and head arts psychotherapies at the Hertfordshire Partnership Foundation Trust. She has held course leader posts at Hertfordshire University (dance movement therapy), Roehampton and Anglia Ruskin Universities (dramatherapy). She currently lectures at Anglia Ruskin University, Cambridge, UK and Codarts, Rotterdam, Netherlands, and practises on a freelance basis. Publications are the edited volumes: *Arts Therapies and Eating Disorders* (1994); *Arts Therapists, Refugees and Migrants* (1998) with Jessica Kingsley Publishers; *Supervision in Dramatherapy* (2008, with Phil Jones), *Dramatherapy and Destructiveness* (2012, with Pete Holloway and Henri Seebohm), and Intercultural Arts Therapies Research (2016, with Margaret Hills de Zarate), all published by Routledge. She has also published numerous articles and chapters, the most recent one on embodiment in dramatherapy (Holmwood & Jennings, 2016).

Dr. rer. medic. Marianne Eberhard-Kaechele is a registered dance-movement therapist, trainer, supervisor, and teaching therapist of the German Dance Therapy Association. She holds the European Certificate of Psychotherapy, is a Kestenberg Movement Profile notator, and ACT trainer. She is a lecturer, researcher, and administrator at the German Sport University, Cologne, department of neurology, psychosomatics, and psychiatry, and teaches internationally in Europe, China, and India. With thirty-five years of clinical experience she now has a private practice in Leverkusen specialising in trauma treatment. She has published over 60 articles and book chapters and is the co-editor of a journal for body psychotherapy and creative arts therapies in Germany. To help establish arts therapies in the German health system she has served on many boards and task forces, and initiated a successful campaign to make Arts Therapies part of a state program to support survivors of incest and institutional violence with additional therapy for up to 10,000€ per person.

Yeva Feldman, is a registered dance movement psychotherapist (ADMP UK), a Gestalt therapist (UKCP) and supervisor (UKCP) with over 20 years of clinical experience working with groups and individuals. Her work with adults with eating disorders has been presented at Confer and other research conferences in the UK and Europe and is described in her chapter "Gestalt and dance movement psychotherapy in adults with eating disorders: Moving towards integration through practice and research" in Payne, H. (ed.) (2017), *Essentials of Dance Movement Psychotherapy: International Perspectives on Theory, Research and Practice*. She co-directs, teaches, and supervises on the MA Dance Movement Psychotherapy Programme at the University of Roehampton and teaches on other Arts Therapies programmes. Additional publications include: "How body psychotherapy influenced me to become a dance movement psychotherapist" in *Body, Movement and Dance in Psychotherapy* journal in 2015 and "Forward" in Unkovich, G., Butte, C. & Butler, J. (Eds.) (2017) *Dance Movement Psychotherapy with People with Learning Disabilities*.

Lisa Lea-Weston is an HCPC registered dramatherapist and supervisor. Lisa was clinical lead for people with profound and multiple disabilities for Devon Partnership NHS Trust and deputy manager of the Arts Therapies Service. Since 2013, Lisa has worked freelance and in private practice and is now specialising in working with children where adoption has broken down or they are in care. Some adult work remains, primarily with those with a diagnosis of DID/trauma. Lisa is the founder of Talking Heads, which provides external supervision to head teachers and SLT nationally to deeply support those that shape children's lives. She has co-established the National Hub for Supervision in Education with Leeds Beckett University. Lisa has presented at conferences in recent years around her work with children and trauma, her own experience of critical illness and creativity, and on working with head teachers through supervision.

David Le Vay is a registered play therapist and dramatherapist. Since qualifying as a therapist in 1992, he has worked extensively with children and young people who have experienced significant loss, trauma, and abuse. David has particular experience, over the last 15 years, of working with a service that provides therapeutic support for children and young people presenting with harmful sexual behaviour. He is currently a clinical partner with The Bridge Therapy Centre and a senior lecturer at Roehampton University on their MA Play Therapy Programme, as well as being an approved BAPT play therapy supervisor and consultant. David has written extensively on his work as a play therapist with children who have experienced complex trauma and recently co-edited a book for Routledge entitled *Challenges in the Theory and Practice of Play Therapy*.

Hayley Marshall is a UKCP registered psychotherapist, and supervisor, with 25 years' clinical experience. She is also a transactional analysis trainer at several TA training centres in the UK. Having worked clinically in outdoor spaces for many years, she has developed a pioneering relational approach incorporating the natural world. She trains and supervises outdoor psychotherapists both in the UK and abroad, and facilitates an advanced outdoor practitioner group in the Peak District. Hayley has co-authored a ground-breaking article on the outdoor therapeutic frame in the European Journal of Psychotherapy in 2010, and has written a chapter on clinical outdoor practice in *Ecotherapy: Theory Research and Practice* published by Macmillan in 2016. She has also written a column on TA outdoor therapy "The View from Here" for *The Transactional Analyst* magazine: www.cen trefornaturalreflection.co.uk.

Jo Salas is the co-founder of Playback Theatre and the founder of Hudson River Playback Theatre in New York State. She has been a core faculty member of the Centre for Playback Theatre and teaches Playback internationally. Her own practice of Playback Theatre includes extensive projects with school bullying, immigrants, and the climate crisis. Jo's publications on Playback Theatre include *Improvising Real Life: Personal Story in Playback Theatre*, now published in ten languages, and *Do My Story, Sing My Song: Music Therapy and Playback Theatre with Troubled Children,* as well as numerous articles, contributions to anthologies, and a TEDx talk "Everyone Has a Story." She created and curates the blog, Playback Theatre Reflects, a venue for thoughtful writing about Playback Theatre.

Prof. Dr. phil. Claire Schaub-Moore CPsychol, AFBPsS, MA DMP is a professor for psychology, chartered psychologist, and counselling psychologist, Associate Fellow of the British Psychological Society, Psychologische Psychotherapeutin, dance and movement psychotherapist, group therapist, trauma therapist, and supervisor. Currently, she works with children, adolescents, and adults in her two practices and as a clinical supervisor for various institutions within the social and health welfare system. For more than fifteen years, Claire has been teaching in HE in Germany, England, and Austria. Furthermore, she has been teaching trauma-pedagogics and traumatherapy for several years. She has conducted several research projects, currently a refugee project, and has published widely.

Dr Julie Sutton is a music therapist and works in a regional adult psychiatry NHS service for patients with severe, complex disturbance. She has over 30 years' experience, has presented, lectured, and been a music therapy and PhD examiner nationally and internationally. Former head of training for Nordoff-Robbins London, among other projects abroad she consulted for the Pavarotti Music Centre in Mostar. A Millenium Fellow, trustee of the British Association for Music Therapy and past editor-in-chief of the British Journal of Music Therapy and vice president of the European Music Therapy Association, Julie is an author of many chapters and articles, including her books *Music, Music Therapy & Trauma* and *The Music in Music Therapy* (2002 & 2014). She is also a qualified psychoanalytic psychotherapist registered with the British Psychoanalytic Council and an executive member of the

Northern Ireland Psychoanalytic Society. She has a private psychoanalytic practice, and is a clinical and research supervisor.

Tara Thornewood is the founding company director of nationally acclaimed Cornucopia Integrated Theatre Company, visiting lecturer at Anglia Ruskin University in Cambridge, and dramatherapist of twenty years' experience, working in forensic psychiatry, adult mental health, and adult learning disability services. Tara is also an actor (including "A Thousand Natural Shocks," Edinburgh Fringe), founding director of "Stories at Home," dramatherapy company working from her narrow boat "home" in Milton Keynes. Tara has previously published in the BADth *Prompt* magazine, reporting on a Forensic Arts Therapies Advisory Group Conference. She enjoys playing with her three children, and trying lovingly to understand her husband of 25 years, and specialising in how our bodies hold psychological and physiological trauma. She is particularly focused on the denial of trauma, and its consequences.

Aileen Webber is a Gestalt and integrative arts psychotherapist (UKCP) working with adults and children in private practice in Cambridge. She is a qualified supervisor of arts-based therapists. Her previous work includes teaching children with a diverse range of special needs. She created and managed a multi-disciplinary enhanced resource within a mainstream school for children with physical, emotional, and learning difficulties, and worked as an advisor and consultant for others working with children with additional needs. She is the author of a book titled: *Breakthrough Moments in Arts-based Psychotherapy* (2017). She is joint creator of a series of therapeutic story start-up books, characters, and scenes, for use in therapy and education (2019).

Gill Westland, MA is director of Cambridge Body Psychotherapy Centre and is a UKCP registered body psychotherapist, trainer, supervisor, consultant, and writer. She is a full member of the European Association for Body Psychotherapy. She is a co-editor of the journal *Body, Movement and Dance in Psychotherapy* and an associate lecturer on the MA Body Psychotherapy programme at Anglia Ruskin University, Cambridge, UK. She is the author of *Verbal and Non-Verbal Communication in Psychotherapy* (Norton, 2015) and has written book chapters and articles on touch in psychotherapy, significant moments of change in body psychotherapy, and the history of body psychotherapy.

Dr Linda Winn is a registered dramatherapist (HCPC). She has extensive experience as a dramatherapist, registered nurse, EMDR practitioner, and psychotherapy supervisor. She currently works as a specialist practitioner in an NHS Perinatal Service where many of the clients have military backgrounds. She has worked with combat veterans and their families and carers for over 35 years. She completed her PhD "The Drama of War, the Theatre of Life – a mixed methods phenomenological case study" at Anglia Ruskin University. This built on her MPhil "Towards a model of dramatherapy for the assessment and treatment of PTSD" (Exeter). Publications include: Winn L. *Post Traumatic Stress Disorder and Dramatherapy* (1994), "Experiential Training for Staff'" in *Arts Therapies and Clients with Eating Disorders* Ed. D. Dokter (1994); Winn, L. and Odell-Miller, H. "Evaluation of the impact and changes in attitudes to military mental health issues for the audience following The Shell Shock Performance" (2018).

Introduction

The idea for this book came out of a cross-professional one day conference in 2016 on the theme of creative approaches to trauma. The theme of going beyond words seemed to be a prominent value in clinical approaches so we, the co-editors, then began a conversation about the interface between creativity, embodiment, and the current neurobiological and neuroscientific literature around trauma.

In considering and unpacking what we see in the field of trauma we identified the following areas:

- environmental trauma – there seems to be quite a prominent area of discourse relating to global warming and endangered species, coastline erosion, etc.
- sociopolitical trauma – ranging from poverty to racism, and war to polarisation of opinion; these factors are not new, but belong to the traumas that are sadly part of human history
- early relational trauma – which ties up with the realm of attachment issues, the impact of postnatal depression, and intergenerational emotional deprivation
- abuse in its many forms (sexual, physical, emotional, and verbal) is fertile ground for trauma and there seems to be an increased readiness to engage with the reality of these many forms of abuse that have previously been cloaked by secrecy
- trauma due to illness, medical procedures, accidents, and crime.

At the same time, there is a developing body of research around the impact and origins of trauma, including presentations which may not initially be named as trauma, but which reveal themselves to be underpinned by trauma (e.g. addiction, challenging behaviours, self-harm).

Our question then was how many therapy approaches to include that operate at this interface. While the recent neuroscientific research has created a climate of radical change in thinking about trauma and clinical interventions, our interest is in how this changing climate is impacting direct work in communities or with clients; in other words, on how theory informs practice.

There are long established arts therapies (art therapy, dramatherapy, dance movement psychotherapy, music therapy) and their child-focused relative, play therapy. In addition to this, we have chosen to give space to embodied psychotherapies – such as, Gestalt, psychodrama psychotherapy, and body psychotherapy – which now include integrative arts psychotherapy. Looking beyond the consulting room, we have included a chapter on Playback Theatre – not a therapy in its own right, but a deeply therapeutic community intervention used globally – as well as nature-based therapy, which honours our context as living organisms in relation to the environment.

Any engagement with trauma work has the potential to take its toll on the practitioner. Hence the inclusion of two chapters; one on therapists dealing with their own trauma through ill-health and one on the significance of an embodied supervisory approach in understanding trauma within clinical settings.

We acknowledge that there are several therapies that are not included and we are also aware of the continuing development of new somatic approaches in the fields of therapy and community engagement.

Trauma is increasingly at the centre of psychotherapeutic, educational, and community practice as well as general health care. Our hope for this book is that it will stimulate and inspire those many practitioners who are working with trauma, whether clinically or in social community settings. We hope also to speak to creative practitioners who may be supported by the theoretical underpinnings explicated in the following chapters.

Students and trainees of psychological, community, and health care disciplines may well benefit from the multiple perspectives on the integration of theory and practice, expressed through the language of different modalities. Case studies shed light on the actual experience of the practitioners in action, taking us into the heart of the therapeutic encounter where there has been trauma.

While this is not a self-help book, those suffering from the impact of trauma may find hope and recognition in this book and may inform themselves of some of the different embodied and creative approaches available.

The book is divided into three parts. In Part I, the focus is on the wider perspective in terms of sociopolitical factors and community engagement.

sissy lykou sets the scene by exploring the sociopolitics of trauma and how experiences that are far beyond people's existing frames of reference eventually transform into trauma, using the example of economic breakdown and subsequent suicidality as well as the impact of embedded societal misogyny. lykou, using an autobiographical example and case study, suggests that one important factor is the degree to which, under pressure, previous self-concepts become incongruent in new circumstances.

Jo Salas, co-founder of the discipline of Playback Theatre, shares with us the value of "enacting testimony." We are invited to witness the application of this creative community method in a variety of global settings in the aftermath of trauma. In each case, personal story is transformed through spontaneous enactment following trauma-informed principles, which Salas explicates.

In Part II, clinical practitioners from a variety of disciplines introduce us to their practice and the theoretical underpinnings of this in relation to clients with trauma histories.

David Le Vay uses the analogy of Keith Jarrett's concert in Köln to unfold the improvisational principles of child-centred play therapy with a traumatised child. He emphasises the therapist's response to the unexpected and unpredictable elements of the therapy session, and the necessity for sensitivity and attunement in building a relationship of trust with his young client.

Following the theme of music, the next chapter takes us to music psychotherapy and Julie Sutton's work with an adult and a young client. Julie describes her specific approach integrating psychoanalytic and music therapy theory. We are introduced to the process of progressing from the experience of timelessness in trauma to temporality, through which the client gains perspective on their reality and the capacity for onward movement.

Gill Westland writes about embodied relating as a core feature of her body psychotherapy approach. She introduces us to a vocabulary of movement and shares with us how she makes use of this theoretical base in her moment-to-moment relating with a client with early developmental trauma.

Anna Chesner writes about trauma-specific approaches to role analytic psychodrama psychotherapy. She emphasises the power of perspective as a particular therapeutic feature of the method. Her case study of a classical psychodrama session with a client with a history of relational trauma demonstrates the therapeutic role of the group, the power of perspective in regulating the intensity of the work, and ultimately the use of non-verbal encounter as an agent of change.

The group theme continues with Yeva Feldman's chapter on Gestalt movement psychotherapy with female clients diagnosed with borderline personality disorder (BPD). Yeva discusses the connection between this diagnosis and trauma experience. She introduces us to the difficulties of engagement that this client group experiences and her sensitive and attuned approach to meeting them where they are; with the main focus of the work being the development of resilience and of embodied resources.

Marianne Eberhard-Kaechele represents the field of dance movement psychotherapy. Practising in Germany, she makes use of movement analysis and draws on a number of theories related to developmental movement to underpin her interventions. Her work on the deconstruction and reconstitution of touch is central. In her case study, we see how blocked feelings and frozen qualities within the client are revived through the use of movement, props, and group.

Linda Winn has developed and researched her own drama-therapeutic model of working with combat veterans. In her chapter, Linda describes the underpinning anthropological theory of Turner's Model of Crisis and the application of this as a paper-based as well as embodied tool. Key to her approach are the use of imagery, metaphor, and aesthetic distance.

Aileen Webber and Sophia Condaris demonstrate an integrative arts psychotherapy approach with an individual client with childhood trauma. The client's connections to her story through her response to Bourgeois' sculpture of a spider is the focal point in this piece of work, where poetry, image-making, and sand-tray are the means for the expression and processing of the unspoken. The authors describe their fluid use of all the art forms in support of the client accessing her story.

Hayley Marshall's chapter focuses on the vitalising and resourcing processes that occur in a nature-based psychotherapy. Through forming a "vibrant alliance" with a "living third," the therapeutic process is infused with further layers of relational immediacy. The natural world acts as co-therapist and offers important non-human resources for systemic regulation. It is also the fluid relational context for therapy. Hayley describes the embodied enlivenment of her client's process and the enhanced possibilities for evoking and transforming early relational experiences and traumas.

Part III takes us from the client focus to that of therapist, team, and supervisor.

Ditty Dokter, Tara Thornewood, and Lisa Lea-Weston's chapter focuses on the impact of secondary traumatisation on therapists facing illness and the importance of creativity in the recovery of resilience. They provide vignettes of their own illness experience and look at the impact on their clients and themselves, as well as the impact of institutional dynamics, clinical supervision, and other forms of support during their illness, treatment, and process of recovery. The importance of creativity in their self-care is considered, especially the survival of hope that creativity may return.

Claire Schaub-Moore's embodied supervision approach is based on psychodynamic theories, movement analysis, and a trauma-informed creative/expressive paradigm. She describes how trauma-informed case supervision is most effective if movement and movement observation are incorporated as genuine aspects in the professional reflection process. Her work takes place in a residential psychiatric context for young people with chronic mental health problems in Germany where she supervises a multidisciplinary team.

We invite you to be as creative as you like in your reading of this book. Whether you follow the journey from beginning to end, taking in the view from different perspectives or whether you dip in and out of those chapters that call you, we hope you find inspiration and companionship in both your professional and personal capacities.

Anna Chesner and sissy lykou
October 2019

Part I

Wider perspective

Chapter 1

Sociopolitical perspectives on trauma in a world in crisis

"The personal is political" revisited

sissy lykou

Sociopolitical trauma is seen as a range of experiences: from political violence against African American and Afro Caribbean people, to the shocks still experienced by those living in Northern Ireland, to the recent refugee crisis, as well as to the ongoing inequalities faced by women. How do society, politics, and history contribute to the creation and continuation of individual, inter-generational, and collective trauma? I will try to form an interdisciplinary understanding of trauma, where the self, in its intrapsychic, interpersonal, and transpersonal guises will be approached via a consideration of the autobiographical, relational, and political body (Allegranti, 2011). All this will be accompanied by the view that an individual's mind-body flow is in relation to past (e.g. the Holocaust), present (e.g. racial and gender discrimination), and future (e.g. the uncertainty of numerous dislocated refugees in Europe).

When I embarked on this venture of first researching the literature and then writing about sociopolitical trauma, I had my direct clinical experience in my mind-body and this informed and shaped my framework, which I can now describe as psychosocial (e.g. Agger, 2001). The psychosocial framework is an attempt to address several observations and issues with the recognition that there is an ongoing and circular interaction between the individual soul and its social environment.

The clinical experience I refer to was in Sure Start children's centres, working with mothers and their children under five years old. Ken Loach's (1994) movie *Ladybird, Ladybird* was my main educator as I attempted to understand, but mainly, to support and fight for the rights of the mothers using the service, who were often in a precarious state, fearing their children would be taken away. In the movie, the main character, Maggie, is a mother of four from an abusive and poverty-stricken background. Social services only check on her and her capacity to bring up her children and offer no emotional support, no opportunities for change or a better life for her and her children. Her four children are taken away from her and she falls into utter despair, pain, and an unbearable sense of loss. She eventually creates a reparative relationship with Jorge, a kind man who accepts her unconditionally and wants to share his life with her. But Maggie is already stigmatised by the social services and society as an "unfit" mother and when she falls pregnant there is a decision that her baby will be taken away as soon as she gives birth. Through my therapy work with the mothers of several groups I was running all over London I witnessed the intergenerational trauma caused by the oppression of women and the underestimation of the impact of the cycles of insecure attachments, as seen also in Maggie's story.

Why, though, did I need to watch the movie in order to educate myself?

This is one of the many examples of gaps and vagueness I have faced in my practice after qualifying and in connection to my own upbringing as a white working-class woman from a small European country, and the limitations that this upbringing carries. Students in psychotherapy trainings are taught that trauma is an outcome of mainly familial aetiology. Although there is a gradual shift in trainings towards a better emphasis on the social and intersectional, there is very little input in terms of understanding the impact of internalised history and of hegemonic structures and ideology (Hollander, 2017). To correct that bias, my writing has a strong element of a personal embodied exploration of my professional position in relation to trauma and its roots and consequences.

How do experiences that are far beyond people's existing frames of reference eventually transform into trauma? How are self-concepts affected when under pressure or new circumstances? How do history and political systems force personal incongruences that lead to trauma? And how seriously do we take our client's despair in relation to existential anxieties, social alienation, and the estrangement from nature?

There is a plethora of writings on intergenerational, transgenerational and cultural trauma and it is not within the scope of this chapter to go through it and explain the differences. But I do want to invite you, the reader, to reflect within your mind-body continuum on the following narrative, allowing at the same time your own history to be present in your reading:

> A war never occurs in just one place or one life. It ripples out in waves of violence that linger – shadows of the official war – lurking behind closed doors, long after the peace treaties have been signed. That war moved from my uncle's psyche [Vietnam war veteran] into mine, through the chambers of my heart, and into the underground trenches of my belly, in the rivers of blood that covered me that day [when he shot himself in front of the author when she was a young girl]. It slowly and invisibly whittles away at my immune system, my memory, my sense of worth, and even my will to survive, until I tried, just like my uncle, to seek out and kill the enemy in myself.
>
> (Matz, 2019)

When I first read Matz's story from the "I" and "we" position that she writes, it became clear to me that when we talk about/work with political trauma, we are not simply dealing with a collection of symptoms, but with an overall destruction of individuals and/or of the social and political structures of a society (Hamber, 2004).

Therefore, in this chapter I am attempting to shed some more light on the notion of sociopolitical trauma as a *"temporal rupture of identity (…), as a wound to the social psyche and body"* (Roberts, 2018, p. 2). In the examples I am using, the defence mechanisms of denial, repression, and dissociation are witnessed and described as processes that modern subjects go through, mirroring biographical, historical, social, and cultural traumas (Herman, 1992; Roberts, 2018).

The nightmares of history and political violence will be part of my reflexive writing that focuses on the betrayal of trust that erases relational ethics and recreates trauma (Audergon, 2004), and on dispossession as a forced – and out of the individual's control – structural dependence on social norms (Athanasiou, in Butler and Athanasiou, 2013).

I have chosen to focus on two specific sociopolitical causes of trauma. The first is in relation to the financial crisis in my native land, Greece, and my dad's death because of it. The second is connected to the #MeToo campaign and the silencing and abuse of women. These causes have shaped me both as a person and as a therapist and, thus, my writing takes a theory-practice way of being perspective rather than a description of a specific psychotherapeutic approach. I hope this also explains the reason why I have not tried to go into any further reflections on all the sociopolitical traumas referred to above.

For confidentiality reasons, the case vignette of the second sociopolitical cause of trauma is a composite based on the material and relational experiences of many different clients, not of an individual.

Not knowing who he was any more: the power of subjectivation[1]

My dad's name was Yiorgos and his surname, Lykos, means "wolf" in Greek. I start with this detail as my dad's story deconstructs the myth of wolves being dangerous to people, and similarly the myth of a working-class father, who lost his business, being a danger to the neoliberal system that demands continuous productivity.

Dad was 59 years and 11 months old when he died, and he was supposed to be able to take his pension when he would become 60 years old. He actually took his life slowly, by not taking his heart medication for many months and storing the boxes at the far back of his wardrobe, in the small flat he had recently moved into after having to leave the family flat with all its memories, comforts, and containment that the latter provided him.

The financial crisis in Greece started in late 2009 and the country has been buried in debt since then. The word "κρίση" (meaning crisis) is in people's everyday vocabulary, political chaos and social turmoil are established parts of the reality, social exclusion and homelessness have increased dramatically, and hundreds of thousands of well-educated and at productive age people have migrated. Unemployment has been significantly associated with the 40 per cent increase of suicide mortality rate (e.g. Basta, et al., 2018), while there is also the hidden number of suicides due to the Orthodox Christian church dominance and their prohibition of burial if someone has taken their life.

My dad's death is one of those hidden suicides. He left no goodbye letter, was not sure when he would die as he took his life in the least painful way he could find, but which also meant that he was carrying this secret on his own for a long time. My sister found him in a coma on the floor of his living room and he managed to stay alive for seven hours. I was not quick enough to reach him, given that I live in London and he lived in Athens. After dad passed away, my sister and I found on his bedside table the letter from the pension office that denied him even a reduced pension simply because he had not paid his contributions for the last year and the owed sum had reached an impossible level for paying due to the interest added every month.

I often have a desperate feeling when I think of dad and how he must have felt having worked very hard his whole life (he had been working since he was fourteen), having contributed to the economy for so many years and then having to silently accept that he would depend on his two daughters – one of whom had migrated to find a better future – for the rest of his life. The image of a man of similar age to dad comes to mind: that man was at an Athens pension office with a blank face, exhausted presence, and curved back. He burst into inconsolable crying when the officer coldly told him that he could not take any pension at all until he paid all the missed contributions. "You can blame the IMF and the Germans," says the officer and the man holds a piece of paper, his body shaking and begging for some mercy. An example of the individual suffering from the cultural trauma of a collapsed economy and a country in social disturbance. Whenever I think of the officer's response, I always feel my body shaking, as if the image of that man, whom I had seen after my dad had passed away, had mirrored all the trauma I had vicariously experienced through dad. McPhillips (2017) postulates that cultural trauma is not something that is done to us but a social process we actively co-construct. This is where my shaking transforms into tension, freezing and immobilisation as expressions of anger and deep disappointment. Hollander (2017) sees neoliberalism as a shaping force of unconscious fantasies, conflicts, and defences and consequently I see the myth of "the IMF and the Germans" making Greek people suffer, as a co-constructed – by the Greek elite, the new-wealth class and corrupt politicians – cultural trauma.

There is a fundamental question for a human who can no longer live their life, who has to accept dependency after a whole life of autonomy: who are you? Athanasiou (Butler & Athanasiou, 2013, p. 75) says in regard to this question "… *its multilayered personal, political, ethical, and affective undertones of impingement, dislocatedness, and even astonishment underlies contemporary debates on recognition.*" "Recognition" is a term of some importance in contemporary debates in philosophy, gender studies, and social theories, as well as in relational psychoanalysis – a debate at the crux of questions about how psychotherapy deals with the wider sociopolitical context. Butler (ibid.) makes the distinction between self-definition and recognition and reminds us of Fanon's notion of the self as socially constituted. In the financial crisis, the "who are you?" has become a form of trauma that bends people, destroys their sense of self and leads them to a regressed state of the Lacanian first stage of relational mirroring with its frag-mented body image – as described in his *Écrits: A Selection* (Lacan, 1977). Con-sidering Winnicott's (1960) notion of "going-on being" under these circumstances and within a traumatogenic culture, I cannot help but think that almost any defence will eventually be subsumed even when trying to maintain it (Hollander, 2017), and that this process takes place in slow motion.

When my dad had to close his coffee shop in June 2013 because he owed quite a lot of money to the tax and pension offices, he started his lonely journey of losing himself in personal private concerns that, although he rationally knew belonged to the collective, he could not, at an emotional level, sustain or make the connection between the collective instability and his own personal crisis. He avoided discussing with us, his daughters, any practical matters as if his unemployment or financial difficulties were personal failings – rather than a social problem (Jones, 2012). Shame would water his eyes, that shame that I can now see as the result of what Layton (2004) calls "normative unconscious"; that denigrates any attachment needs, that over-evaluates agentic capacities and only values attitudes such as competition and self-reliance.

Depression finally took away from dad any sense of agency in the world. He would socialise only with my sister and sometimes with my mum, his mum, and his brother. His physical health declined and on two occasions he fainted but dismissed the incidents and refused to go to the doctor.

Dad used to express his love by holding my hands and caressing them. I learned from him that words are not necessarily the best way to express one's self. The last time I saw him, almost a month before he died, he held my hands while I was in the stranded train to the airport and he was on the platform and I remember my strong feeling of belonging to our family and the values of love, care, and sharing. But what had happened to dad's belonging? Rozmarin's (2017, p. 476) definition of belonging resonates with me: "… *(it) is a crucial aspect of human experience*" where one feels "*singular within shared pluralities*" (emphasis in the original). In retrospect, I imagine that dad's sense of belonging had become alienated in his embodied trauma of loss of his position in the society, of his autonomy and hope for life; in other words, in his political incapacitation (Athanasiou, 2019).

"*Trauma (…) devastatingly disrupts (…) the sense of stretching along from the past to an open future*" (Stolorow, 2019) and indeed the financial crisis, which has dominated the whole world, deprives individuals from their embodied existential hope that there can be any meaningful change for the better in the future (Ratcliffe, 2015). This kind of psychosocial trauma alters the individual's bodily felt sense of "I can" (Stolorow, 2019) and leads to a pretence that crushes the soul (Schuck, 2019).

I will conclude this part of my chapter with Jessica Benjamin's poignant words that bring the performative aspect of witnessing into politics and society: "*The social recognition of trauma is not only healing for individuals, it pro-motes agency and gives weight to ethical considerations within the social dis-course*" and "*… it calls us to be witnesses (…), a container for its* (the trauma) *examination*" (Benjamin, 2014, as cited in McPhillips, 2017, p. 143).

The silencing of women

In Pina Bausch's *Viktor* (first performed in 1986) a woman in high heels, long and elegant green dress, and a heavy coat storms onto the stage and shouts first at a mirror and then at a silent man who looks at her: "Why are you looking at me? Leave me alone." She repeats this with remarkable intensity while her body leans forwards, and her head leans backwards; giving an image of her being off balance. I catch myself kinaesthetically empathising with this *fragilisation* (Lacan, 1977) of the performer's body and, with uncontrollable tears, I try to hold what feels more like a collective, a more long-term pain among women. But I swiftly realise that I could not have felt more alive in this time of connection ...

Finkel (1991) comments on *Viktor* and the several scenes with women suffering but presenting themselves in nice clothes or smiling while in pain, that Bausch is aware of and presents sadness and beauty and the ways these can be linked. Servos (2008, p. 122) on the same piece: "*It describes a woundedness which must be maintained and withstood, which does not let up till it has reinstated the happiness of being entirely at one with ourselves.*"

What does the shouting woman represent in today's society and in previous eras in a world that has proclaimed "*the war on women*" (Lloyd-Roberts, 2016)?

Valerie is in her mid-forties, a politically active middle-class British woman who accessed therapy when the #MeToo campaign was at its peak. Her first words were "I now feel allowed to voice my story and not be scared that I will be silenced." When I heard Valerie saying this, Lorde's (2017, p. 2) words came to my mind "*I was going to die, if not sooner then later, whether or not I had ever spoken myself. My silences had not protected me.*" And I could deeply sense Valerie's fear of revealing to her own self, first of all, the trauma she had gone through; the danger (and power) of transforming her language into language and action (Lorde, 2017).

Lorde (2017), Solnit (2017), and Olsen (1965/2003), all felt like my female ancestors holding my hand while, I, as a therapist, was trying to understand and process the sociopolitical obstacles we, women, have been facing throughout history. Solnit (2017, p. 45) describes clearly the silencing process women undergo and fight against: "*Silence is a burden that belongs or belonged to most of us, though some are more loaded with it than others, and some have become experts and geniuses in how to shove it aside, drop it, disown it.*"

When Valerie enquired about therapy, she had already broken up with her former male partner of five years. This was her first long-term relationship and, in a way, an idealised one as the disappointment caused by the several short-term previous relationships had governed her sense of self and had projected an expectation of perfection in this most recent one. The main reason that brought her to therapy, though, was that she still felt scared of accidentally seeing her former partner anywhere in the city she lived in. This caused her an ongoing sense of alertness, anxiety, and fear. She also suffered from insomnia, as she kept ruminating about the debt she had accumulated due to the legal costs in the process of her trying to protect herself from her former partner. The lack of legal aid (see the financial cuts in legal aid in the UK affecting people's safety and women's reporting of abuse) exacerbated her sense of being unprotected in this "dominated by men world" (her words). She lived in a constant precarious financial state as her work in the arts field had fluctuations of income and employment, so the debt felt like a long-term trap. Here I would like to draw a brief connection with my dad's story and the impact of the financial crisis worldwide and within all generations. Valerie wanted to face the ghosts of the past that would often govern her dreams, would make her feel agitated with the slightest suspicion that a man in front of her could have been her former partner, and would become a loud and intimidating voice telling her that she is not enough. It gradually became apparent that in the long-term relationship she was subjected to emotional abuse and twice she was beaten up for reasons that she could still not understand. She had internalised a shrinking image of herself based on her former partner's words that he had created her, that she needed to behave in certain extroverted ways other-wise she was an embarrassment for him, and that her work was not important (her former partner worked in finance). Her thinking would go into repetitive loops of shame and self-blaming; "Why didn't I see what I was going through? Why did I trust him for so long? How could I not respect myself, me a politically active and inde-pendent woman who is aware of women's rights?"

Her trauma was highlighted by conversations with friends and acquaintances, when she would be asked why she didn't do anything about it or why she stayed with him. Valerie found these questions abusive, like another kind of silencing, as she knew that these were the questions she constantly asked her own self. Abuse within intimate relationships does not appear like a sudden attack and as such the shock is not immediate but a trapped feeling that lingers within the mind-body and gradually dominates the individual.

There are several issues within the questioning of Valerie's actions by others. First, we see the societal lack of patience in listening to the other's pain, and the consequent jumping to conclusions, opinions, questions, as a way of finishing the conversation or silencing the speaker, in touch with her pain. In *Regarding the Pain of Others,* Sontag (2003) accuses the privileged – in whatever situa-tion – for their distant engagement with the other's pain and postulates that this attitude is an act of dismissing politics. Privilege tends to limit or obstruct one's imagination; being part of the dominant group means that one sees themselves and not the others (Solnit, 2017).

Then we have the issue of horizontal hostility when these questions come from women. Does Valerie, and every woman who has been traumatised by an intimate relationship, have to deal with the fertilised violence among women, a phenomenon based on the fragmentation of women's groups that try to band together but who inevitably internalise the patriarchal control over them? And where can feminism fit in such exchanges? Ahmed (2010) talks about *feminist consciousness* not as a simple consciousness of gender but that of "... *the vio-lence and power that are concealed under the languages of civility and love*" (Ahmed, 2010, p. 86). It is, indeed, a big step to realise in what world you live, rather than the one you thought you were in, and when the injustice of the world you live in is pointed out to you via fellow women's stories, then you are forced to make this step; it ceases being a choice.

Another issue is when these questions are posed by men. Then, the vicious cycle of *"feeling wrong, being wrong; being wronged"* (Ahmed, 2017) dominates the woman who is consequently silenced and plays the well-known game of "keep calm and carry on."

In my work with Valerie I tried to examine with her the costs of recognition within a struggle of survival (Butler, 2015) both within her former relationship, as well as within her wider circles and our society. Her fidgety, uncomfortable, shrinking presence was understandable in a world occupied by male privilege.

"Feminism can begin with a body, a body in touch with a world, a body that is not at ease in a world, a body that fidgets and moves around, (...) as things don't seem right," says Sarah Ahmed (2017, p. 22). With this in my own mind-body, I invited Valerie into a journey of disentangling this shrinking, of expanding in the space and fighting back gendering that defines which bodies can take up space. Grounding from within rather than searching for it outside was, also, a focus in our embodied movement work.

A generic definition of the term *kinesphere* is that of the space we occupy when interacting, relating, being in the world, and the imaginary boundary of it. When I asked Valerie to first move within her "bubble" that would symbolise her kinesphere, and to then draw her experience, I saw a pattern I have seen several times in my work with women survivors of domestic abuse: small, hesitant, and bound movements that reached out and soon after were drawn back, close to the body and a drawing that concentrated on the bottom part of an A3 piece of paper, taking up only one third of the page space. Through movement improvisation we, as a dyad that represented several relationships in Valerie's life, tried to bypass the repression that dominated her life in the five years with her former partner and to diminish any repetitions. I would also extend a consistent invitation for emotive gestures that came as free associations to the thoughts and reflections we were exploring. These relational movement sequences enabled Valerie to start going through a process of redefining her subjectivity and, in a way, claiming a visceral presence on the stage of her life and that of the world (Climenhaga, 2009).

I mentioned earlier the notion of "grounding from within." This is a movement approach I have developed borrowing elements from Frank and La Barre's (2011) notion of "embodied history," the human connection to nature and the myth of Persephone; all these in relation to the impact of any kind of abuse on a woman. "Grounding from within" was the result of my intense embodied responses to my female clients' stories of physical, emotional, and sexual violence. Ahmed again (2017, p. 21–22): *"... feminism begins with sensation [...]. Feminism often begins with intensity [...]"* and feminism has definitely shaped my way of being in therapeutic relationships.

Let me now explain the connection of "grounding from within" with the myth of Persephone. Persephone is the goddess of Spring and nature, inseparably connected to earth and the ground; that ground that also took her away from her life, and her mother, and friends. Hades bursts through a crack in the earth and abducts Persephone. The myth is also known as "the rape of Persephone" and symbolises the suddenness and disempowerment of such an act from a man against a woman. Similarly, in my approach, I aim to work with the symbolism of disempowerment and the sudden deprivation of power when trauma occurs. By supporting my clients to visualise their verticality no matter what the ground feels like, I aim to build up with them, and in them, a strong sense of the spatial pulls that relate to the end poles of up and down (Hackney, 2002). As opposed to body approaches that mainly emphasise the downwards, grounding movement, this simultaneous upwards and downwards pull, well known to dancers, is more effective when the ground is unstable or when just standing still is not an option. This supports the embodiment of the client's congruent subjectivity. A visual demonstration of my approach can be seen in my drawing in Figure 1.1.

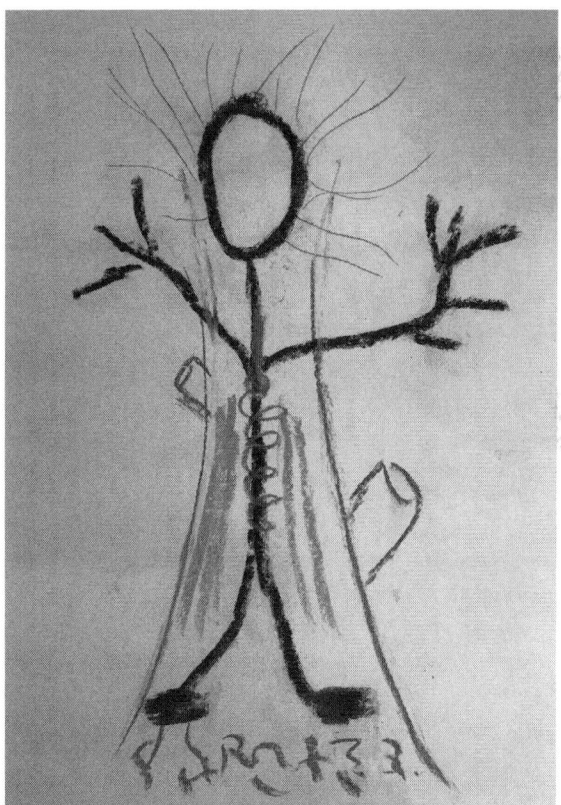

Figure 1.1 Grounding from within

Women, as eternal Persephones, carry within their subjectivities "incorporative memories" (Fuchs, 2012), memories that shape our bodies-for-others, like carriers of social symbols, cultural inscriptions that trap our bodies. In this way, a woman's trauma of abuse can (wrongly) be justified as something that happens, given that women throughout all generations have been carrying the guilt of being responsible or that they should not talk about what happened to them and keep going with the wound(s) paining them forever. What is fundamentally a socio-political issue, is pointed out as an individual issue, and it becomes a political issue again through the processes of blaming and silencing. Finally, the incorporative memory becomes "traumatic memory" (ibid.).

Therefore, the interplay between the private and the public worlds are part of the work therapy offers to women survivors of abuse and with the 1970s motto *"the personal is political"* (Hanisch, 1970) we can restore some inner connections and regain power through speaking the unspeakable (Herman, 1992).

It is not my aim to unfold a specific case and go through the steps of Valerie's therapy, thus the limited history information and very specific mentioning of my therapy approach. The use of case material was the frame for looking more closely at the trauma women can carry, how this demonstrates itself in therapy, and how it can then be viewed and processed from an embodied-politicised intersubjective perspective.

Afterthoughts

I would like to conclude my sharing and reflections with the consideration of two concepts as these could be applied in the therapy field: collective reflexivity and consciousness (e.g. see consciousness of racism or feminist consciousness in Ahmed, 2010). I see these two concepts as the means for restoring connections between the public and private worlds (Herman, 1992), in the consulting room or wherever else therapy movements (can) take place.

Finally, trauma and mobilisation can be seen and felt together in therapy as an attempt for our clients to gain back their reflexive subjectivities (Butler, 2015). Butler, Gambetti, and Sabsay (2016) suggest that we think of vulnerability and resistance together, and I would add that we (both therapist and client) experience them as our vertical tensions between two poles – an up and down continuum with tension as well as synchrony – that keep reminding us of our presence in the world in crisis. After all, these are two concepts that can help us develop "… *a different conception of embodiment and sociality within fields of contemporary power*" (ibid., p. 6).

Note

1 A Lacanian term that describes the process that creates the subject. Hollander (2017) adds that it is an uncritical identification that reproduces foundational values and institutional arrangements both in the realm of ideas, as well as in everyday behaviours.

References

Agger, I. (2001). Psychosocial assistance during ethnopolitical warfare in the former Yugoslavia. In D. Chirot & M. Seligman (Eds.), *Ethno-political warfare: Causes, consequences and possible solution* (pp. 305–318). Washington, DC: American Psychological Association.

Athanasiou, A. (2019). Formations of political-aesthetic criticality: Decolonizing the global in times of humanitarian viewership / Athena Athanasiou in conversation with Simon Sheikh. Curating after the Global. MIT Press. Retrieved from www.academia.edu/40344594/Formations_of_political-aesthetic_criticality_Decolonizing_the_global_in_times_of_humanitarian_viewership_Athena_Athanasiou_in_conversation_with_Simon_Sheikh.

Ahmed, S. (2010). *The promise of happiness*. London: Duke University Press.

Ahmed, S. (2017). *Living a feminist life*. London: Duke University Press.

Allegranti, B. (2011). *Embodied performances: Sexuality, gender, bodies*. Basingstoke, UK: Palgrave MacMillan.

Audergon, A. (2004). Collective trauma: The nightmare of history. *Psychotherapy and Politics International*, 2(1), 16–31.

Basta, M., Vgontzas, A., Kastanaki, A., Michalodimitrakis, M., Kanaki, K., Koutra, K., *et al.* (2018). Suicide rates in Crete, Greece during the economic crisis: The effect of age, gender, unemployment and mental health service provision. *BMC Psychiatry*, 18. Retrieved from https://bmcpsychiatry.biomedcentral.com/articles/10.1186/s12888-018-1931-4.

Butler, J. (2015). *Senses of the subject*. New York: Fordham University Press.

Butler, J. & Athanasiou, A. (2013). *Dispossession: The performative in the political*. Cambridge, UK: Polity Press.

Butler, J., Gambetti, Z., & Sabsay, L. (Eds.) (2016) *Vulnerability in resistance*. London: Duke University Press.

Climenhaga, R. (2009). *Pina Bausch*. London: Routledge.

Finkel, A. (1991). Gunsmoke. In R. Climenhaga (Ed.) (2013), *The Pina Bausch sourcebook: The making of tanztheater*. London: Routledge.

Frank, R. & La Barre, F. (2011). *The first year and the rest of your life: Movement development and psychotherapeutic change*. New York: Routledge.

Fuchs, T. (2012). The phenomenology of body memory. In S. Koch, T. Fuchs, M. Summa, & C. Müller (Eds.), *Body memory, metaphor and movement* (pp. 9–22). Amsterdam, Netherlands: John Benjamins.

Hackney, P. (2002). *Making connections: Total body integration through Bartenieff fundamentals*. New York: Routledge.

Hamber, B. (2004, April). The impact of trauma: A psychosocial approach. Keynote address to the A Shared Practice – Victims Work in Action Conference, N. Ireland. Retrieved from www.brandonhamber.com/publications/pap-trauma1.htm.

Hanisch, C. (1970). The personal is political. In S. Firestone & A. Koedt (Eds.) *Notes from the second year: Women's liberation – major writings of the radical feminists*. New York: New York Radical Women.

Herman, J. (1992). *Trauma and recovery: The aftermath of violence – from domestic abuse to political terror*. New York: Basic Books.

Hollander, N. (2017). Who is the sufferer and what is being suffered? Subjectivity in times of social malaise. *Psychoanalytic Dialogues*, 27(6), 635–650.

Jones, O. (2012). *Chavs: The demonization of the working class*. London: Verso.

Lacan, J. (1977). *Écrits: A selection.* New York: W.W. Norton.

Layton, L. (2004). Relational no more: Defensive autonomy in middle-class women. *Annual of Psychoanalysis,* 32(1), 29–42.

Lloyd-Roberts, S. (2016). *The war on women: And the brave ones who fight back.* London: Simon & Schuster.

Loach, K. (Director). (1994). *Ladybird, Ladybird* [Motion picture]. UK: Film4.

Lorde, A. (1977/2017). *Your silence will not protect* . London: Silver Press.

Matz, L. (2019). Fishing for fallen light. *Stillpoint: Digital Magazine in the Eye of the Storm,* 2. Retrieved from https://stillpointmag.org/articles/fishing-for-fallen-light/.

McPhillips, K. (2017). "Unbearable knowledge": Managing cultural trauma at the royal commission. *Psychoanalytic Dialogues,* 27(2), 130–146.

Olsen, T. (1965/2003). *Silences.* New York: Feminist Press.

Ratcliffe, M. (2015). *Experiences of depression: A study in phenomenology.* Oxford: Oxford University Press.

Roberts, J. (2018). *Trauma and the ontology of the modern subject: Historical studies in philosophy, psychology, and psychoanalysis.* London: Routledge.

Rozmarin, E. (2017). Immigration, belonging, and the tension between center and margin in psychoanalysis. *Psychoanalytic Dialogues,* 27(4), 470–479.

Schuck, C. (2019). Toward an age of certainty and uncertainty. *Society for Humanistic Psychology Newsletter,* July. Retrieved from www.apadivisions.org/division-32/p ublications/newsletters/humanistic/2019/07/future-survival.

Servos, N. (2008). *Pina Bausch: Dance theatre.* Berlin, Germany: K. Kieser Verlag.

Solnit, R. (2017). *The mother of all questions: Further feminisms.* London: Granta publications.

Sontag, S. (2003). *Regarding the pain of others.* London: Penguin Books.

Stolorow, R. & Atwood, G. (2019). *The power of phenomenology: Psychoanalytic and philosophical perspectives.* London: Routledge.

Winnicott, D.W. (1960). The theory of the parent-infant relationship. *The International Journal of Psycho-Analysis,* 41, 585–595.

Chapter 2

Enacting testimony

Trauma stories in Playback Theatre

Jo Salas

Trauma is the experience of dreadful terror and helplessness in the face of a threat that is beyond the capacity of the individual to cope with, and from which she or he is unable to escape. "The essence of trauma is that it is overwhelming, unbelievable, and unbearable" (van der Kolk, 2015, p. 195). It may result from a single incident – an accident, an episode in war, a natural disaster – or from experiences that continue over years, like domestic abuse. It may occur at any age from infancy on, or even earlier, in cases of transgenerational trauma. It may be consciously remembered, or not. For some people the immediate impact of the trauma fades over time, without clinical help. Painful echoes may remain permanently, to be stirred up from time to time by new stresses or life changes. For other trauma sufferers, because of the severity or duration of the trauma or other complicating factors, normal life becomes impossible in the face of horror and its damage to the soul.

Recovery from trauma, whether spontaneous or assisted by clinical treatment, is generally acknowledged to require a sequence of stages, described by Judith Herman (1992, p. 155) as "a gradual shift from unpredictable danger to reliable safety, from dissociated trauma to acknowledged memory, and from stigmatised trauma to restored social connection." She and other theorists of trauma (e.g. van der Kolk, 2015; White and Epston, 1990) emphasise the central role of storytelling after the essential first phase of establishing safety. At first, storytelling is likely to be a private narration, however incomplete or disorganised, of what happened. Later comes a more public storytelling that can restore the traumatised person's sense of meaning and connection to society. "In the telling, the trauma story becomes a testimony," Herman writes. "Testimony has both a private dimension, which is confessional and spiritual, and a public aspect, which is political and judicial" (1992, p. 181).

For van der Kolk (2015), Herman's stages of storytelling represent only one "avenue" of trauma healing. Another avenue is the use of pharmaceuticals or other technologies. And a third is "allowing the body to have experiences that deeply and viscerally contradict the helplessness, rage, or collapse that result from trauma" (van der Kolk, 2015, p. 3). While primarily exploring methods that can address the physiological effects of traumatic stress – muscle tension, breath, heart rate, brain functioning – van der Kolk also acknowledges that most people need some combination of these approaches. Levine's approach also emphasises somatic experience: "[T]rauma is something that happens in the body. We become scared stiff or, alternately, we collapse, overwhelmed and defeated with helpless dread. Either way, 'trauma defeats life'" (Levine, 2010, p. 31).

Playback Theatre and trauma

This chapter is about how Playback Theatre, a mostly non-clinical resource, can contribute to the integration of trauma both individually and societally through stories, artistic embodiment, and the call to imagination – another key element in trauma healing, according to van der Kolk: "Without imagination there is no hope, no chance to envision a better future, no place to go, no goal to reach" (2015, p.17). Although adaptable for use in therapeutic settings, Playback Theatre is not primarily a therapeutic modality. Its main use is in the wider community with participants who are not diagnosed with mental illness or disorders. Based on the universal desire to tell one's story, the need to know beyond doubt that it has been heard, and the yearning to hear the stories of others, Playback Theatre has been adopted worldwide in contexts that include theatres, classrooms, refugee camps, staff retreats, and prisons, as well as in therapeutic treatment.

The basic format of Playback Theatre is this: a volunteer relates a personal experience and others act it out on the spot. Other stories follow, building a dialogue of images and themes. In performances, stories are told by audience members and enacted by a team of trained improvisers including a musician, with the facilitation of a "conductor." A performance typically includes short dramatised reflections of brief statements from audience members as part of a warm-up process, followed by three or four longer stories and a closure. In this unscripted theatre, the artistry lies in the performing team's ability to transform raw experience into aesthetically coherent, emotionally meaningful theatre, with distilled language and expressive movement – all based on their empathic comprehension of the teller's story.

Playback also frequently takes place in groups such as training workshops, professional development sessions, or therapy groups, without a designated performing team. Instead, one or two leaders guide participants in enacting stories for each other, using the same basic format. A heightened ritual atmosphere prevails even in the most informal or intimate settings, with a distinct arrangement of the space, a consistent sequence in time, and the attentive, authentic demeanour of the conductor and actors. This ritual aspect is fundamental in Playback Theatre, creating a strong and flexible container for whatever stories may come.

Playback is a theatre of everyday life. It seeks to lift up the stories of ordinary people by embodying them in aesthetic form. It welcomes stories of joy, delight, discovery, and humour as much as stories of sorrow and struggle. At the heart

of Playback Theatre is the rich complexity of real lives, along with the conviction that as social beings we long to know and learn from each other's life
experiences. Fulfilling this longing is healing in itself, not in a clinical sense, but
in the wider sense of affording insight, ontological meaning, affirmation, a sense
of belonging, and community cohesion. A performance or workshop is fundamentally a collective event. Although the utmost attention is paid to each individual voice, the overall meaning comes from the interwoven story of the group
and the sense of connectedness that it engenders.

Playback Theatre's effectiveness in addressing trauma belongs mostly to the
third stage of Herman's formulation, when trauma sufferers are ready to give
"testimony" in order to rebuild their sense of belonging to the community, to
gain validation, and to claim their right to justice in cases where they were
wronged. When this testimony is embodied in creative action the teller sees her
story from the outside, perhaps for the first time. She and other watchers
respond kinaesthetically to the movements, voices, and interactions of the
actors. The teller knows *with her body* that she has been heard. She, as well as
audience members, may be "moved" in a literal sense, as they respond to the
action onstage and are drawn imaginatively into the teller's story – breath
changes, bodies lean forward, laughter or tears may come.

The recognition of these integral elements – storytelling, embodiment, artistry, and imagination – has led to Playback's use with communities coping with
collective and individual trauma in the wake of a natural disaster, political or
personal victimisation, and other significant hardships.

In a women's prison

The other members of Hudson River Playback Theatre and I are in the yellow-
painted recreation room of a medium-security women's prison, two hours north
of New York City on the Hudson River. It is World AIDS Day. About 60
women troop in wearing dark green prison garb – young, middle-aged, a few
elderly. Most are African American, with others who appear to be Latina or
white. This day is a sombre anniversary for people whose lives have been
shadowed by HIV/AIDS. We are prepared for stories of grief, loss, shame. M,
the social worker who is our liaison, is a necessary presence: the women know
and trust her, and we trust her too. She will be available for whatever follow up
might be needed. This is our fourth visit for AIDS Day. Some of the women
remember us from previous times and they greet us warmly. Others, sentenced
in the past year, keep their distance.

We start with a song. The women join in, the newcomers' reserve melting
quickly. In response to our warm-up questions they tell us about missing their
loved ones – far away children, family members who have died.

I invite a volunteer to come to the teller's chair onstage and tell a longer story
from her life. Hands go up immediately. I choose a woman who spoke up earlier. The others call encouragement as she makes her way to the stage area.

"Brianna, right?" I say as she sits down beside me. "Where does your story begin?" Brianna was in the audience the year before and she knows the ritual. Perhaps she decided ahead of time to tell her story tonight. She launches into it with a bold statement: "I got AIDS." Brianna looks at the audience as if in defiance. Although HIV/AIDS has touched almost everyone's life one way or another, having the virus oneself carries stigma here and is normally kept secret. The audience is now silent except for a murmur or two of support. Brianna continues. Her story is about how she became infected as a teenager. It is a horrendous story of rape, incest, violence, and abandonment. Her defiance evaporates and her voice becomes almost inaudible. I have to repeat her words so that others can hear. To my right, the social worker draws her chair nearer. Brianna chooses one of the three actors to play herself in the story. The actors and I know that we need to be very careful in this enactment – to embody her story accurately enough that it is meaningful to the teller, without over-whelming her. Brianna has chosen to tell her story tonight. She has judged that this is a safe place and time to reveal not only her AIDS status but also how she was desperately wronged by her brother and her family. Despite her agency, however, she is still vulnerable and fragile.

Accompanied by quiet keyboard chords, the actors begin the enactment. They depict the violence with the slightest of movements, a far from literal portrayal. Even so, it's too much for the teller. She lowers her head, unable to watch. I call out for the actors to pause so that I can check in with her. Would she like us to stop? No, Brianna says, she wants to see her story. But it's hard. With her agreement we decide to continue with a series of short forms embodying feelings, not characters or events. Brianna watches this time, tears falling, her hand gripping mine, but nodding in assent. The actors pause and look towards her, as they always do at the completion of a scene. Brianna nods again and lets out a breath. Then she faces the women in the audience, several of whom are also in tears. "But I want to say, look, here I am, they didn't kill me," she says. The audience breaks into loud applause and cheers. Brianna goes back to her chair. The women sitting on each side of her hug her, one after the other.

Brianna had lived with her terrible memories and their life-threatening con-sequences for some years. Time, if not therapeutic help, had allowed her to metabolise her traumatic experience to the point that she was ready to tell her story in front of peers, through the vehicle of the theatre that we offered. She received the affirmation that she hoped for: the other women, instead of rejecting her, showed their respect, empathy, and moral indignation at what had happened to her. Even so, the theatrical depiction of her story had to be carefully titrated, in Levine's term (2010), allowing Brianna to apprehend her story at the degree of intensity that she was able to tolerate. Every gesture by the actors, every interaction, would have its echo deep within her body and her brain. Too much could harm her. Too little would disappoint her. The cor-rectly judged potency would help her to take another step in her journey of integration.

There was also an altruistic element to Brianna's story. In the prison community, other women looked up to her. By telling her story, she challenged the stigma that clung to HIV/AIDS, lightening the burden of others who were afraid to reveal they were infected.

Stories of natural disasters

Playback Theatre teams have sought to support communities coping with trauma following the 2005 tsunami in southern India, Hurricane Katrina in New Orleans, the earthquake and tsunami in Fukushima, Japan, and other natural disasters. Though each event is different, disaster-related trauma has characteristics that are distinct from other kinds of trauma, even other collective trauma. Natural disasters happen with little or no warning. They disrupt the previously normal lives of vast numbers of people, sometimes with hundreds or thousands of casualties. The immediate crisis itself is time limited – a matter of hours or days, though chaotic, and life-threatening consequences may last for years.

Playback post-disaster teams have sometimes been composed of people who are themselves part of the affected community (as was the case in India and New Orleans). In other situations, the team has come from outside the disaster area but is culturally congruent (as in Japan after Fukushima). NOLA Playback Theatre – NOLA stands for New Orleans, Louisiana – was born in the aftermath of Katrina:

> A little over seven months after the "levee breaks" disaster of August 2005 and two months into the life of our company, NOLA Playback Theatre performed at a popular New Orleans theatre festival ... I was still living out of our emergency trailer fifty miles north of our flooded home with my husband, toddler, baby, two rescued cats and the contents of our attic ... I opened the event by asking for a show of hands as to who was back in their homes and who was still living out of a FEMA trailer or somewhere else. Most of the room was still displaced.
>
> (Juge Fox, 2013, p. 22)

When the Playback team is based elsewhere, it is necessary to develop relationships with the people in the disaster region, networking and communicating over time until there is a trusting partnership that can work together on this most sensitive of projects. In the absence of such patiently developed relationships, a well-intentioned Playback team runs the risk of parachuting in on a rescue mission and possibly creating harm rather than healing, or – more likely – failing to have any impact at all when the hoped-for audience simply does not show up.

Following Fukushima, the Yokohama-based company PlaybackAZ wanted to offer Playback Theatre to survivors in the ravaged area, 700 kilometres away. They knew they needed a local partner, but months went by without finding the right connections. They gave up the idea of visiting and instead offered fundraising performances and events for volunteers returning from Tohoku

(Munakata, 2013). They also used this time to educate themselves about collective trauma following a natural disaster, as well as learning the specific details of the Fukushima disaster, a complex event that included a major earthquake, a devastating tsunami, and the deadly release of radiation from the nuclear power plant.

Eventually, a man with connections to Tohoku came to one of their performances for volunteers and saw the potential for his community. Eighteen months after the earthquake, a group of four company members made their way to Tohoku. They stayed for three days and carried out four performances for volunteer helpers and local people. Kayo Munakata describes a story told by an old woman in one of the shows:

> A [childhood] story about school excursion. Mothers used to make big rice balls for their lunch. A friend of the teller dropped her rice ball and she lost all her lunch. So the teller shared her rice ball. She gave half of it.
>
> It was just a small story.
>
> But it apparently reflected their sudden tragedy and a spirit of friendship and of supporting one another.
>
> (Munakata, 2013, p. 21)

With the performers' sensitive, aesthetic reflections and their acceptance of whatever stories were offered, the atmosphere deepened. Later in the show another elderly woman told a story about her losses in the tragedy, releasing intense emotion – her own and the audience's – and a flow of further stories.

This Playback team was open to whatever stories the audience members chose to tell, whether addressing the disaster directly or in metaphor, or even recalling apparently unrelated experiences. A key principle in Playback Theatre is emergence. The stories are not curated. If we have established an atmosphere of respect, authenticity, and inclusivity, we trust that the stories offered are the stories that need to be told and will contribute organically to the overall tapestry of the event. This is the process now known as narrative reticulation (Fox, 2018), where stories weave together to create meaning that transcends any individual story. A story that seems slight, indirect, or even humorous – dropping one's lunch on the ground; the comical annoyance of hitting a pothole on a New Orleans street – are nevertheless playing their part in allowing a traumatised community to feel its connections, its strength of history, its pain, and its resilience.

Stories of political oppression

Political oppression inevitably creates trauma, tragically common in today's world, with millions of people affected by war, terrorism, extreme poverty, and climate change. Playback Theatre teams have sought to support groups of refugees or displaced persons in the UK, the Netherlands, Germany, Angola, and elsewhere (Glover, Mitchell, Stedmon, Fairlove, & Brown, 2016; Salas, 2011). Such groups face the same responsibilities as in post-natural disaster interventions of building relationships and cultural congruence before attempting to enact stories. Political awareness and analysis become essential preparation.

Wasl, a Playback Theatre group in Lebanon, provides performances to trau-matised communities including Syrian refugees (one person in four in Lebanon is a refugee), victims of human trafficking, and young men whose poverty made them vulnerable to being recruited by ISIS:

> We had a big project, 16 performances, within a closed community, more of a ghetto, that is considered the main pool of Lebanese fighters for ISIS in Syria and Iraq. [After a show where grieving mothers told their stories] a very silent guy who usually attended the shows but never shared came to us to thank us. The next day the organiser of this project from the same area gave us a call to thank us, telling that the guy who came to greet us and a few of his friends who were supposed to join the war in a few days, deci-ded after hearing and watching the stories of the two mothers that they would rather be in prison than leave their loved ones with such pain and sadness. So they went to the military and delivered themselves. In prison their recruiters couldn't reach them so they were safe and alive.
>
> (Wardani, personal communication, 18 April 2018)

This work is extremely challenging for the performers, who feel under threat because of their insistence on foregrounding the voices of victims of war rather than those of so-called martyrs and heroes. Emotional strain and vicarious traumatisation are risks for any Playback ensemble working in situations of intense crisis. As well as self-education about history and context, groups must also strengthen themselves emotionally by telling their own stories in the safety of a rehearsal, giving each other generous support, finding effective ways of relieving tension, getting outside support if needed, and taking care not to commit to more performances than they can sustain.

During Hudson River Playback Theatre's eight-year series of bilingual per-formances for immigrants in upstate New York, stories of life-threatening danger, loss, and suffering, told with intense emotion, were common (Salas, 2008). Many audience members had fled dead-end poverty and often violence in hopes of building something better for their children. Some had come close to death crossing river and desert. Women had been raped. Children had been taken from parents, close relatives lost. Living in the United States, their hard-ship was not over: they now faced discrimination, isolation, separation from extended families, and the threat of deportation.

Participants seemed impelled to tell border-crossing stories and wept as they watched their stories brought to life. Often the audience wept with them. "It makes us sad to remember, but happy to see it," said one woman. Their stories were public testimonies –to each other, to their children who were often present, and to those who represented the majority culture, sometimes just the Playback

team, sometimes other members of the community as well. The immigrants tes-
tified to their hardship, to their vision, courage, and resilience, and to their
identity as the newest community of immigrants in a nation of immigrants.

Such trauma stories, as in other contexts of political oppression, are not
simply expressions of individual suffering. The teller "speaks not only for personal salvation – they speak with political intent" (Rivers, 2013, p.15). Citing
research indicating that potentially traumatising events are far less likely to lead
to PTSD when survivors "interpret their experience through a strong ideologi-
cal framework" (ibid., p.16), Rivers describes how Playback Theatre supports
this kind of positive framing:

> Playback Theatre with its inbuilt potential for consciousness raising, meaning-
> making and community mobilization, holds promising possibilities for the
> reinforcement of certain protective factors. When a teller shares their account
> and sees it enacted within a communal setting, the teller is able to establish a
> sense of coherence around their experience – especially where their story is
> framed within the broader context of civil resistance.
>
> (Rivers, 2013, p. 16)

It is also essential to remember that all lives, even those of people in extreme suffering, contain love, beauty, triumph, and humour. A critic claimed that stories
about "good" aspects of life showed "avoidance" behaviour (Rivers, 2013, p. 16).
On the contrary, such stories are a sign of resilience and a Playback performance
should embrace them, for the audience's sake and for their own. Farah Wardani
(2018) in Lebanon also writes about enacting joyful, affirming stories, like preparing for a traditional wedding or celebrating success at school. And they often invite
tellers to imagine a more hopeful future, enacting those images as well.

Trauma stories in therapeutic settings

In therapeutic settings, Playback Theatre's collective and performative nature
lends itself best to the later stages of trauma recovery. When survivors are ready
to share their story with others, the contained ritual of Playback can provide a
welcoming space. For example, Playback Theatre in a residential treatment
centre gave traumatised children a chance to reveal some of their stories to
peers, mitigating isolation and prompting empathy:

> Sharelle had been in one of the Playback therapy groups for several weeks. In
> the fifth session she told about a memory from when she was two years old.
> Finding her playing alone outside on the porch, her stepfather had picked her
> up and dangled her over the railings, chuckling as she screamed in terror for
> her mother inside. The mother didn't come, either not hearing or not caring.
>
> I asked Prue [co-leader] to play Sharelle's stepfather. Sharelle chose waif-
> like Aimee to play herself and Olly to be her mother. To my surprise, Olly

agreed readily to this cross-gender role. He was a quiet boy, self-conscious about a bad stammer. They acted it out. I could see Olly struggling with the desire to come and help Aimee/Sharelle as she screamed in fear. But he stayed true to the story.

"Yeah," said Sharelle when they'd finished. "Felt like that."

Watching the story was freckle-faced Herman ... "I wish the mom had come out and helped her," he said, his hands pressed to his throat as always when he spoke. "I felt bad for Sharelle." I hadn't heard this kind of expression of pity and identification from him before.

(Salas, 2007, p. 113)

Our staff team carried out both classroom performances and therapy groups, where children enacted stories for each other. The worst abuses that these children had suffered, including sexual victimisation, extreme violence, even torture, did not emerge in Playback Theatre. Most could not yet speak of those horrors even in the privacy of a one-to-one session with a psychologist. They instinctively knew which stories could be told in Playback, and which could not. On one occasion, this judgement broke down. A child dealing with a very recent trauma offered it as a story in a classroom performance: his young uncle had been murdered just weeks earlier. Mayhem ensued. For other children in the room, the topic was far too raw. Thanks to quick-thinking teamwork we were able to recover the situation, but it was a lesson in the danger of trying to enact a story that is not yet ready to be a testimony, in the presence of others watching with their own traumatised eyes (Salas, 2007).

Unexpected trauma stories

Trauma is a part of life and may come up in any Playback Theatre event including public performances, though more likely in a training workshop where participants are together for several days. As practitioners, we need to recognise the signs of a trauma story, usually signalled by the content and the intensity of emotion. We need to understand that this story is being told as "a transition toward the judicial, public aspect of testimony" (Herman, 1992, p. 221). We have to attend to not only the teller's wellbeing, but also that of the audience and the performers. Advanced training in Playback Theatre now includes attention to dealing with trauma both in these occasional stories and in collective trauma situations.

Ideally, we are alert also to a wider story: even the most personal story takes place in a societal context. It may be relevant – and healing – to reflect that reality in the enactment, whether it is the prevalence of domestic abuse, the harms of racism or poverty, or the ravages of addiction. Although a teller may focus only on her family tragedy as she speaks about her addicted son, those listening, including the performing team, are also thinking of the current opioid epidemic. It is appropriate and constructive to depict that awareness in the enactment.

Conclusion

Playback Theatre's inherent aspects of collective storytelling, embodied and artistic distillation, and the call to the imagination can help transform painful, overwhelming memories into meaningful stories that survivors can tell to themselves and to others. It can allow suffering individuals and communities to reclaim their humanity and their hope.

In the public or semi-public settings that are Playback's most common context, practitioners do not need to be therapists. However, they do need to be well grounded in basic Playback skills, and to be mindful of several factors including these:

- the effectiveness of a Playback show for a traumatised audience depends on relationships that have been carefully developed prior to the event, especially if the team members are not part of the affected community
- ideally, these relationships are sustained over time, as with NOLA Playback's ongoing engagement with the New Orleans community, or a Palestinian team's practice of staying in a village for several days to help with daily tasks and exchange learning (Rivers, 2013)
- offering Playback too soon in the recovery process can be harmful or ineffective: both tellers and audience members need to be ready for public testimony
- trauma stories may convey resilience and solidarity alongside personal pain and need not be pathologised
- with an audience that has survived or is currently dealing with significant trauma, stories that might seem unrelated or "light" are in fact part of the process of asserting resilience[1]
- using Playback's variety of forms, enactments need to be "titrated" in order not to overwhelm a teller
- trauma stories may emerge in any Playback context

With attention to these considerations, the Playback stage – informal, accessible, ritualised –can indeed embrace stories of trauma, contributing to individual and societal recovery.

Note

1 However, if a collectively traumatised audience offers *no* direct stories of the trauma in the course of an event, it may indicate that using Playback is premature, or that the Playback team is not sufficiently prepared to hold these stories – which the audience will unfailingly sense.

References

Fox, J. (2018). The theory of narrative reticulation: A brief description. Unpublished article.

Glover, K., Mitchell, A., Stedmon, J., Fairlove, A., & Brown, A. (2016). And I felt as if I'm home you understand, with my people. *IPTN Journal*, 2(1). Retrieved from www.iptn.info/?a=doc&id=362&lang=[mb_lang].

Herman, J. (1992). *Trauma and recovery: The aftermath of violence—from domestic abuse to political terror*. New York: Basic Books.

Juge Fox, A. (2013). NOLA Playback Theatre & *un*performing disaster in New Orleans. *Interplay*, 13(2), 22–23.

Levine, P. A. (2010). *In an unspoken voice: How the body releases trauma and restores goodness*. Berkeley, CA: North Atlantic Books.

Munakata, K. (2013). Before you saw a hill here; now you see the ocean: How Playback Theatre serves communities in crisis. *Interplay*, 13(2), 19–21.

Rivers, B. (2013). Playback Theatre, cultural resistance, and the limits of trauma discourse. *Interplay*, 13(2), 15–18.

Salas, J. (2007). *Do my Story, sing my song: Music therapy and Playback Theatre with troubled children*. New Paltz, NY: Tusitala Publishing.

Salas, J. (2008). Immigrant stories in the Hudson Valley. In Solinger, R., Fox, M., & Irani, K., (Eds.), *Telling stories to change the world* (pp. 109–118). New York: Routledge.

Salas, J. (2011). Stories in the moment: Playback Theatre for building community and justice. In Cohen, C., Varea, R., & Walker, P. (Eds.), *Acting together: Performance and the creative transformation of conflict*, Vol 2, (pp. 93–123). New York: New Village Press.

van der Kolk, B. (2015). *The body keeps the score: Brain, mind, and body in the healing of trauma*. New York: Penguin Books.

Wardani, F. (18 April2018). Personal email communication.

White, M. & Epston, D. (1990). *Narrative means to therapeutic ends*. New York: W.W. Norton.

Part II

Clinical perspectives

Chapter 3

The unplayable piano

From discord to harmony: trauma, play therapy, and the power of the non-verbal

David Le Vay

Introduction

On 24 January 1975, shortly before midnight, the acclaimed jazz pianist Keith Jarrett prepared to play to a 1400 capacity audience in the opera house in Cologne, Germany. The audience were expectant. Jarrett himself was exhausted after a long drive from Zurich. He wore a brace to alleviate his acute back pain and had hardly slept or eaten prior to the concert. The concert itself had been organised by Vera Brandes, who at seventeen years was Germany's youngest concert promoter and, as requested by Jarrett, had arranged for a Bösendorfer 290 Imperial concert grand piano to be made available for the performance. However, a few hours before he was due to play, Jarrett discovered that the opera house staff had mistakenly brought out the wrong Bösendorfer piano, a practice piano used for rehearsal only. The intended Bösendorfer was not available and so Jarrett found himself confronted with a piano that was in such poor condition that he deemed it to be "unplayable."

It required several hours of hasty hard tuning to get the piano close to a basic state of playability but even so the upper registers were thin and tinny due to the worn-out felt on the hammers, the base register was weak and dull, the pedals did not work properly, and the piano itself was too small for its sound to fill the large space of the opera house. Jarrett initially refused to play, but was finally persuaded by the young and increasingly desperate Vera Brandes. The performance by Jarrett was almost entirely improvised, opening with a delicate phrase of five notes that echoed the call bell that had played in the lobby moments earlier (interestingly, Jarrett said later that he was unaware of this – as if it were something almost unconsciously intuitive) and from these five opening notes flowed a piece of music, the Köln Concert, that went on to become the best-selling solo album in jazz history and the all-time best-selling piano album with sales of over 3.5 million.

Playing within the constraints of the piano, Jarrett avoided the upper registers and kept within the mid-range of the keys, giving his playing a gentle, ambient tone. The lower base registers had to be played harder than usual to generate enough sound to project to the back rows of the hall and at times he stood, hammering at the piano with a mesmeric intensity. On the recording, Jarrett can be heard vocalising as he plays; groaning, goading, and chanting as he wrestles a performance from his instrument, and his feet can be heard stamping on the pedals with a percussive force that punctuates the concert. Like much of Jarrett's playing, it is as much physical theatre as it is musical performance. Ultimately, it was a sublime, seminal performance created in the moment, from the moment. As Jarrett (2014) himself said, *"what happened with this piano was that I was forced to play in what was – at the time – a new way. Somehow I felt I had to bring out whatever qualities this instrument had."*

So why am I telling you this story? Firstly, I should say that my daughter's birth was accompanied by the Köln Concert, so I have to declare a degree of author bias. I know the piece intimately, almost note for note. Secondly, as well as being a dramatherapist and play therapist, I am also a jazz pianist and am hence inherently interested in the correlation between musical improvisation and the playful process of child-centred therapy. As an arts and play therapist, the story of the Köln Concert resonates in many ways. It makes me wonder about the experience of the unexpected or the unpredictable; the constraints we might feel within ourselves, the children we work with or indeed within the relationship. It makes me wonder about how, as therapists, we manage chaos, mess, unpredictability, the unplayable child one might say, and how we find a point of connection. The notion of harmony from discord, the search for balance and equilibrium, is something that in essence lies at the very heart of the therapeutic process. And faced with the unplayable, we also have to confront our own anxiety about the unknowable. As the dramatherapist Sue Jennings (1995, pp. 132–141) would say, "stay with the chaos and meaning will emerge" and for the child-centred play therapist it is the oft quoted mantra of "trust the process." Or as Jarrett himself said, faced with his unplayable piano and an expectant 1400 audience in the Cologne Opera House, *"my sense was ... I have to do this. I'm doing it. I don't care what the piano sounds like. I'm doing it. And I did"* (2014). In the absence of words we cannot know what a child's experience of trauma sounds like, looks like or feels like. So we have to find a playful point of creative connection where meaning can indeed begin to emerge and the child's story can be told.

Within this chapter, I aim to explore the process of child-centred play therapy from the somewhat unusual perspective of both play therapist and jazz improviser, taking my cue from Jarrett's experience of his unplayable piano and the metaphorical lessons we might draw from this story as we engage therapeutically with troubled children in the playroom. Furthermore, I will aim to explore the role of the nonverbal process of working with children who have experienced complex trauma and abuse; my central thesis being that an ever-emerging neurobiological awareness and understanding of the impact of trauma is supporting what, as arts and play therapists, we have intuitively known for some time; that this work more often than not sits in a space beyond words (Harris, 2009; van der Kolk, 2015).

Periodically throughout this chapter I will draw on a brief vignette from my clinical play therapy practice, with the aim of illustrating key aspects of the discussion in hand. All case material used is both anonymised and disguised. That said, if anyone thinks that perhaps they do recognise any of the material discussed I trust that it can be read in the spirit in which it was written and intended; with the utmost respect for those involved.

> Stuart was twelve years old with a background of chronic early neglect, domestic abuse and developmental trauma. Made subject to a care order, he experienced a succession of foster placements all of which broke down due to his challenging and often aggressive behaviour. Deemed unplaceable (certainly unplayable) Stuart was moved to a children's home with a therapy service on site where he attended weekly play therapy sessions over a two year period. Stuart's expectation was of a world that was dangerous and unpredictable and his predominant narrative identity – his self-story – was one of rejection and it was this sense of feeling fundamentally unwanted that he constantly sought to recreate. Indeed, it was the one thing that was familiar to him.

Child-centred play therapy: a brief overview

Child-centred play therapy (CCPT) is a developmentally appropriate therapeutic approach that employs play as the primary mode of intervention (Axline, 1947/1989; Cochran, Nordling & Cochran, 2010; Landreth, 1991). It is a developmentally appropriate approach in the sense that CCPT fundamentally recognises play as the primary, natural language of the child; the way in which children communicate, explore, and understand their world. In this sense, the play therapist seeks to *meet* the child; to find a point of playful connection that is congruent with the child's developmental stage. CCPT is child led and is based upon the belief that, through the process of play and within the context of an empathic, non-judgemental therapeutic relationship, the child has the capacity to communicate and begin to make sense of the complex and confusing feelings that can be the result of problematic life experiences.

Historically, the notion of play being utilised as a therapeutic intervention has its roots in the work of the early psychodynamic pioneers of child psychotherapy such as Klein (1932), Lowenfeld (1935), and Anna Freud (1927), who recognised the symbolic, unconscious, and primarily non-verbal nature (and value) of the process of children's play. The specific child-centred model of play therapy is rooted in the client/person-centred psychotherapy model established by Rogers (1951) and developed further by Axline (1947/1989), who drew upon the person-centred approach to develop a clear, theoretical, and principled framework for the practice of non-directive play therapy (NDPT).

The central premise within CCPT maintains that children possess the innate tendency towards self-actualisation (Maslow 1962), in other words an instinctive drive towards growth and balance, given the right psychological conditions. To this end, CCPT holds the role of the therapeutic relationship as the central agent of change, facilitated by the core conditions of empathy, unconditional positive regard, congruency, and genuineness (Axline 1947/1989; Landreth 1991). In regard to terminology, the terms *non-directive* and *child-centred* tend to be used somewhat interchangeably to describe this model of play therapy, acknowledging the key influences of both Axline and Rogers. The distinction between these terms is, I would suggest, largely semantic, the nuanced emphasis being upon the use of self and how one positions oneself within the therapeutic relationship. For the sake of continuity and consistency I will use the term CCPT throughout.

> Highly dysregulated, Stuart was one of the frightened/frightening, the lifetime legacy of developmental trauma, and his window of tolerance was minimal. It took him many weeks before he felt safe enough to spend any length of time in the playroom. For some reason there was a music system in the playroom – it was shared space – and for the first few weeks Stuart would arrive 'armed' with a CD and a defiant glint in his eye. The CD was usually some kind of fearsome drum and bass or "gangsta rap" which he would play at a deafening volume. As a strategy, it was an effective defence against therapy and the use of words. The windows rattled and shook, the air crackled, and each week Stuart waited to see what I would do. Would I tell him to leave, turn the music down or turn it off? Would I end the session? Stop seeing him? Words were impossible, thinking was hard, but the fear and aggression was palpable. And each week I did nothing except to sit with him in this aural maelstrom; experiencing it together. After a while, when he realised that I was not going to do as he expected, Stuart would turn down the volume himself to a bearable level. This was an early turning point in the work, which saw Stuart testing my capacity to contain this initial assault upon my senses but which also led to his own capacity to self-regulate; to turn down the background noise of his trauma to a point where we could begin to connect.

Play therapy, developmental trauma and the trouble with words

Play therapy, alongside the allied arts and creative therapies, is becoming increasingly recognised as an effective and evidence-based therapeutic approach for working with children and young people (Bratton, Ceballos, Sheely-Moore, Meany-Walen, Pronchenko & Jones, 2013; Lin & Bratton, 2015; Schumann, 2010; Stulmaker & Ray, 2015). Furthermore, the arts and play therapies are becoming increasingly informed by an ever-developing understanding of neurobiology and neuroscience, not least within the context of complex, developmental trauma.

Emerging evidence (Glaser, 2000; Klorer, 2008) suggests that trauma experiences are stored primarily in the non-verbal and pre-verbal regions of the brain's right hemisphere. Further to this, evidence suggests (van der Kolk, 2000) that at the time of original trauma experience (and associated extreme hyperarousal) there is a significant reduction in activity in the left side of the brain and those regions responsible for language and declarative memory. More specifically, fMRI scans indicate a reduced function – in effect a shut down – in the hippocampus region, an area that plays an important role in the consolidation of information from shorter to longer term memory (Hart & Rubia, 2012; McLaughlin, Sheridan, & Lambert, 2014; Teicher, Anderson, & Polcari, 2012). As is also now well documented (Hull 2002; van der Kolk, 2000) neuroimaging studies of people experiencing PTSD indicated a decreased level of functioning within the Broca's area (the region of the brain linked to speech production) during exposure to traumatic script.

So what does this all mean? Firstly, it needs to be acknowledged that sustained empirical evidence regarding the neurobiological impact of psychological trauma is limited, particularly so, the evidence in relation to children, so we have to be cautious about generalisation. That said, the emerging research (Hull, 2002; van der Kolk, 2000) does indicate a neurobiological context within which traumatised individuals, and I would suggest particularly children and young people, struggle to verbally articulate their traumatic experiences, particularly when experiencing intense levels of anxiety and emotional dysregulation. Added to this is the fact that children's trauma is often experienced at a pre-verbal level, for example through in-utero exposure to toxic substances, i.e. drugs and alcohol, traumatic birth experiences, early separation, medical intervention, and the developmentally traumatic impact of neglect and abuse in the early, formative years of their lives. So we have the combination of neurobiological impact and potential cognitive impairment, both of which may well contribute to difficulties with verbal engagement.

Of course, this is just part of the picture. Children who have experienced traumatic abuse also experience overwhelming levels of shame and stigma; significant barriers to verbal engagement. Abuse more often than not takes place within a context of secrecy; children are silenced and abuse remains unspoken. Children referred into therapy carry with them very dominant personal narratives around shame, self-blame, internalised guilt, and intense experiences of fear and threat. Within the play therapy room, silence and all that this means can be a salient feature of the child's experience and process. As David Crenshaw says (2010, p. 4), silence is "a poignant presence by virtue of the absence of spoken words." The challenge for the therapist is to understand the context and meaning that silence has for the child. Is it about neurological, trauma-induced shut down, in the sense that there are no words that can communicate the child's experience? Or is it about shame, secrecy, and the child's experience of being silenced?

Alternatively, the capacity to join the child in a process of silent, reflective therapeutic reverie can be intensely powerful, evoking Winnicott's (1958) notion of the capacity to play alone – in the presence of another. More often than not, this is about how as therapists we manage our own anxiety in the absence of words and resist the impulse to *act* rather than *be*. I am often reminded of the fable of the Elephant and the Frog. The story tells of an elephant that got hold of a particularly tasty looking palm leaf but accidently drops it into a muddy pond. The more the elephant thrashed and splashed around in the pond the muddier the water became and the harder it was for the elephant to find the palm leaf. Nearby, sitting on a stone, a little frog watched the proceedings with a curious interest. "Be still" the frog said after a while in a quiet voice. But not listening, the elephant continued to thrash around in the muddy water looking for his leaf. "Be still" whispered the frog again. The elephant kept on splashing. "Be still" the frog said for a third time. Exhausted through his effort, the elephant finally stops and listens. "What did you say?" the elephant asked the frog. "Be still, breathe and wait for a moment" the little frog said. And as the elephant remained still and breathed and waited, the water in the pond began to clear as the mud slowly settled. "Now look down" said the frog. The elephant looked down. There was the palm leaf. He reached down and pulled it out with his trunk and happily began eating again. Sometimes as therapists we need to stop, pause, breathe, and allow for space and silence to notice the importance of what is happening in front of us.

So the emergent picture is of a complex dynamic between neurological, developmental, and emotional/psychological factors that all contribute to the difficulties children and young people have in articulating their experiences of trauma and abuse. As Gil (2006) reminds us, the combination of all these factors can result in a natural resistance to talking about their abuse and so the critical stage in therapy is that of engagement – finding a way to connect with a child that does not feel too emotionally overwhelming. Words, at this stage, can feel too intrusive. Gil (2006) continues, "the right hemisphere of the brain is the most receptive to non-verbal strategies that utilise symbolic language, creativity and pretend play. Thus, art, play sand and other expressive therapies may be necessary components of trauma treatment" (ibid, p. 68).

> As the weeks progressed, Stuart would take to hiding under the table, in the corner of the playroom, with a blanket over him. There was a hole in the blanket that he looked through, so he could see me but I couldn't see him. He would instruct me to shut my eyes and stand in the middle of the room where he could see me (although I confess to cheating and squinting a little). Sometimes twenty minutes would pass without words. Sometimes, from the safety of his blanket, Stuart would throw things around the room, sometimes hitting me with them. I would talk aloud to myself; wondering what the noises were? Where were they coming from? What might happen next? Was I safe? I talked about feeling alone and vulnerable in the middle

of the room and worried that I might be hurt. In the silence, I talked to myself about Stuart under the table; that maybe it felt safer under there; that he could see me but I couldn't see him. Sometimes I wondered if this was what it was like for little Stuart ... when he lived at home. Stuart did not have to say anything. Non-verbally, he was very powerfully communicating his feelings and letting me know about his world.

A playful window of tolerance

To return for a moment to the metaphor of the Köln Concert and the unplayable piano, the fact that Jarrett had to keep within the mid-range of the keyboard, the playable range, while avoiding the unplayable lower and upper registers of the piano, brings to mind the notion of the Window of Tolerance (Ogden, Minton, & Pain, 2006) and the importance of enabling children to stay within their own emotionally tolerable mid-range. The upper register of Jarrett's piano was harsh and tinny, the lower range deep, rumbling, and inaudible; an aural evocation of the hyperaroused or hypoaroused response of the dysregulated child. Most play therapists will have encountered the unplayable child; the child who is either too chaotic or too frozen to be able to playfully engage, or the dissociative child who has learned to survive through disconnection.

Allied to this model of the Window of Tolerance, Polyvagal Theory (Porges, 2011) proposes three key evolutionary developmental stages of the autonomic nervous system; mobilisation, immobilisation, and social engagement. Mobilisation links to the hyperaroused child and the fight-or-flight behaviours dependent upon the sympathetic nervous system. Immobilisation relates to the primitive, dissociative hypoaroused state of the parasympathetic response. The state of social engagement is one of calm, communicative reciprocity within which both verbal and non-verbal relational interaction can facilitate a process of positive therapeutic engagement. This is the integrated window of the child's experience and children who are enabled to remain within their 'window' and tolerably connect with their experiences in an integrated way are able to engage in a process of energised, creative, and dynamic play.

At the heart of this process is a therapeutic relationship that feels safe and contained. Therapy is a relational experience, as of course is abuse and trauma, and subsequently children's experience of the world is of a place that is frightening, unpredictable, and dangerous. In this sense, the initial intimacy of the therapeutic encounter may feel, in itself, overwhelming and, to an extent, intolerable for some traumatised children and so the beginning stages of the process are all about safety, containment, and a relational point of connection that enables children to stay within their mid-range, window of tolerance. As Allan Schore states (2009, p. 130), the therapeutic relationship enables clients to "re-experience dysregulating affects in affectively tolerable doses in the context of a safe environment, so that overwhelming traumatic feelings can be regulated and integrated into the client's emotional life."

Sometimes Stuart would play in the sandtray, presenting as much younger than his chronological years. Invariably, his repetitive stories involved cars that had crashed and become trapped in the sand – immobile. He would bring in a rescue vehicle, attach it to the back of the trapped car and pull it to safety to be repaired at the garage. Sometimes the vehicles would not attach properly and Stuart would become agitated, evocative of his own experience of feeling unattached and disconnected. Later, looking through his social services file I found pictures he had drawn when he was five years old of him trying to rescue his mother from being physically assaulted by his father. As his sand-play continued over the weeks, I was encouraged by the arrival on the scene of a policeman, batman and other benign rescuers that seemed to symbolise some sense of moral order. Again, in the absence of words but in the context of a therapeutic relationship, Stuart was showing me how his world use to be – and how it could be.

Connections, attunement, and the playful improviser

Jarrett's mirroring of the house signal bell at the very beginning of the Köln concert is interesting, as if he needed to engage with something external to access an internal place of creative contemplation – a state of reverie one might say. Like a process of therapeutic attunement, facilitating emotional regulation, Jarrett intuitively took his external cue and used it to move away from the back pain, the hunger, and tiredness to a place where he could meet and connect with his unyielding, resistant instrument free from judgement and frustration. Finding a point of initial contact, a way to meet the child, is the beginning of the therapeutic encounter and in many ways sets the tone of the relationship. A little like Jarrett and his unplayable piano, Landreth (1991, p. 156) says of the first time of being in the child's presence, "I experience a challenge of what will we, the child and I, be able to create here?" What does this child need, Landreth asks, the challenge being to find a point of connection accepted, both uniquely and unconditionally. Jarrett had to ask himself that very same question; what does this piano need in order for it to perform to its best potential and what do I need to do to facilitate this process?

The notion of empathic attunement lies at the heart of the therapeutic relationship. Attunement, as the very word suggests, is about a harmonious synchronicity (Hart 2018). In keeping with the musical metaphor of Jarrett and his piano, it is about resonance, rhythm, and spontaneous creative reciprocity. There is something magical about the act of attuned pitch and frequency that can see one string begin to vibrate and come to life when matched with the frequency of another. In play therapy, this is about gesture, tone, proximity, a shared affect that brings therapist and child in *contact* with one another; a harmonious, playful connection. As Stern (1985, p. 142) suggests, attunement is the "performance of behaviours that express the *quality* of feeling of a shared affect state." So, this is not so much about a fusing or a mirrored imitation but more about the felt, intuitive sense of being empathically experienced and understood by another. Within play therapy, we are more often than not working with children whose relational needs have not been met. For children who have experienced trauma and abuse, their early attachment and attunement experiences are invariably problematic, distorted, and discordant.

It is also important to acknowledge that while the Köln Concert was a spontaneously improvised piece of music, it was not without form or structure. Jarrett of course performed frequently, in a variety of contexts and styles, so would have developed an internal framework of sorts from which he could scaffold, build, and develop his musicality – a kind of internal repertoire from which he could draw. His playing that night would have been informed by a rich depth of patterned phrasing or intuitive characterisation honed over many years of experience and experimentation; a secure base from which he could explore, knowing he had a place to return to. This does not detract from the improvisational nature of Jarrett's playing, but simply provides parameters or a framework within which it can exist. This is of course analogous to the play therapy process, the therapist's character and style developed through experience and informed by the core therapeutic qualities of empathy, congruence, and unconditional positive regard. The theory underpins the practice, not in a way that restricts or inhibits the natural playfulness and curiosity of the therapist but rather provides the security of foundation and form. Jarrett is also an accomplished classical pianist and in this sense it is his very knowledge of the theory that allows him to move away from it, just as the unconsciously competent play therapist is enabled to engage in playful improvisation within the playroom.

Peter Elsdon's (2013) examination of the Köln Concert suggests particular phrasings that Jarret uses when he gets stuck, "rescue manoeuvres" that enabled him to creatively negotiate the less travelled paths that he might unexpectedly find himself on. At times, as play therapists, we often encounter uncharted territories; the unpredictable, the chaotic, and the unfamiliar. As we follow the child's lead there is by definition an "improvisational edge" to our work where at times we are working within the realm of unconscious competence, where both therapist and child are working on the fringes of the uncomfortable. Perhaps this is the place where the work gets done? Some might refer to this as the liminal space (e.g. Harris, 2009); a transitional, transformative, unknown place that lies somewhere "betwixt and between" and sits on the threshold between the conscious and unconscious. Within improvisational jazz this is a place of dynamic, exciting, and sometimes risk-taking creativity, and I would suggest that the same could be said for the process of non-verbal, child-centred play therapy.

After two years, towards the end of our sessions, Stuart would create shocking images of baby dolls, bound and gagged with tape. He would soak them in water and then tell me about living at home and when his father and his friends use to stand and urinate over him. It took a long time, but going at Stuart's own pace he eventually got to a point where he could move from the nonverbal to the verbal and find a way to begin to communicate his traumatic experiences safely. More than anything, he had begun to find a way to play – no longer the unplayable child. The projective power of his sessions was intense, often overwhelming, to the point that I still carry a little piece of him within me.

Trauma, then, may well at times render a child unplayable and as a therapist one has to be alert to the signs that might indicate a child's stuck, post-traumatic play, for example the absence of spontaneity, joy, affect, and indeed playfulness. But I would suggest that all children have the capacity – the potential – to be playful, and the challenge for the therapist is to find a creative point of connection and therapeutic presence to allow that potential to emerge, as Jarrett did with his unplayable piano. The nature of interpersonal trauma brings paradoxical challenges around emotional and physical proximity; the child that wants to be close but does not want to be near, and this can feel a little like walking a tightrope as one endeavours to simultaneously maintain both a critical distance from and a critical connection to the child. The non-verbal element of play therapy is fundamental to this. Words are rarely enough. Just as the improvisational jazz musician seeks the magical space between the notes, the improvisational therapist needs to be alert to the space between the words.

As Keith Jarrett himself once said, "jazz is there and gone. It happens. You have to be present for it. That simple."

References

Axline, V. M. (1947/1989). *Play therapy*. London: Churchill Livingstone.

Bratton, S. C., Ceballos, P. L., Sheely-Moore, A. I., Meany-Walen, K., Pronchenko, Y., & Jones, L. D. (2013). Head start early mental health intervention: Effects of child-centered play therapy on disruptive behaviors. *International Journal of Play Therapy*, 22(1), 28–42.

Cochran, N. H., Nordling, W. J., & Cochran, J. L. (2010) *Child-centred play therapy: A practical guide to developing therapeutic relationships with children*. Chichester, UK: John Wiley.

Crenshaw, D. (Ed.) (2010). *Reverence in healing: Honoring strengths without trivializing suffering*. Lanham, MD: Jason Aronson.

Elsdon, P. (2012). *Keith Jarrett's The Köln Concert*. Oxford: Oxford University Press.

Freud, A. (1927). Introduction to the technique of child analysis. In *The writings of Anna Freud*. New York: International Universities Press 1974.

Gil, E. (2006). *Helping abused and traumatised children: Integrating directive and non-directive approaches*. New York: The Guilford Press.

Glaser, D. (2000). Child abuse and neglect and the brain – a review. *Journal of Child Psychology and Psychiatry*, 41(1), 99–116.

Harris, D. A. (2009). The paradox of expressing speechless terror: Ritual liminality in the creative arts therapies' treatment of posttraumatic distress. *The Arts in Psychotherapy*, 36, 94–104.

Hart, H. & Rubia, K. (2012). Neuroimaging of child abuse: A critical review. *Frontiers in Human Neuroscience*, 6, 52.

Hart, S. (2018). *Brain, attachment, personality: An introduction to neuroaffective development*. London: Routledge.

Hull, A. M. (2002). Neuroimaging findings in post-traumatic stress disorder. *The British Journal of Psychiatry*, 181, 102–110.

Jarrett, K. (2014). Pianist Keith Jarrett: The story of the Köln Concert. Interview with Don Heckmann. Retrieved from www.grammy.com/grammys/news/pianist-keith-ja rrett-story-k%C3%B6ln-concertgrammy.com. The Recording Academy.

Jennings, S. (1995). Playing for real. *International Play Journal*, 3, 132–141.

Klein, M. (1932). *The psycho-analysis of children*. London: The Hogarth Press and The Institute of Psycho-Analysis.

Klorer, G. P. (2008). Expressive therapy for severe maltreatment and attachment disorders: A neuroscience framework. In C. A. Malchiodi (Ed.), *Creative interventions with traumatized children*. New York: Guilford.

Landreth, G. (1991). *Play therapy: The art of the relationship*. Levittown, PA: AD Taylor Francis.

Lin, Y. & Bratton, S. C. (2015). A meta-analytic review of child-centered play therapy approaches. *Journal of Counseling and Development*, 93(1), 45–58.

Lowenfeld, M. (1935). *Play in childhood*. New York: Mac Keith Press distributed by Cambridge University Press. 1991.

McLaughlin, K. A., Sheridan, M. A., & Lambert, H. K. (2014). Childhood adversity and neural development: Deprivation and threat as distinct dimensions of early experience. *Neuroscience and Biobehavioural Review*, 47, 578–591.

Maslow, A. H. (1962). *Towards a psychology of being*. Princeton, NJ: D. Van Nostrand.

Ogden, P., Minton, K., & Pain, C. (2006). *Trauma and the body: A sensorimotor approach to psychotherapy*. New York: W.W. Norton.

Porges, S. W. (2011). *The polyvagal theory: Neurophysiological foundations of emotions, attachment, communication, and self-regulation*. New York: W.W. Norton.

Rogers, C. R. (1951). *Client-centred therapy*. Boston, MA: Houghton Mifflin.

Schore, N. L. (2009). Right-brain affect regulation: an essential mechanism of development, trauma, dissociation, and psychotherapy. In Fosha, D., Siegel, D., & Solomon, M. (Eds.), *The Healing power of emotion: affective neuroscience, developmental and clinical practice*. New York: W.W. Norton. 2009.

Schumann, B. (2010). Effectiveness of child-centered play therapy for children referred for aggression. In J. Baggerly, D. Ray, & S. Bratton (Eds.), *Child-centered play therapy research: The evidence base for effective practice*. Hoboken, NJ: Wiley.

Stern, D. (1985). *The interpersonal world of the infant: A view from psychoanalysis and development psychology*. London: Karnac Books.

Stulmaker, H. L. & Ray, D. C. (2015). Child-centered play therapy with young children who are anxious: A controlled trial. *Children and Youth Services Review*, 57, 127–133.

Teicher, M. H., Anderson, C. M., & Polcari, A. (2012). Childhood maltreatment is associated with reduced volume in the hippocampal subfields CA3, dentate gyrus, and subiculum. *Proceedings of the National Academy of Sciences*, 109, 563–572.

van der Kolk, B. (2000). Posttraumatic stress disorder and the nature of trauma dialogues. *Clinical Neuroscience*, (2)1.

van der Kolk, B. (2015). *The body keeps the score: Mind, brain and body in the transformation of trauma*. London: Penguin Books.

Winnicott, D. W. (1958). The capacity to be alone. *International Journal of Psycho-
Analysis*, 39, 416–420.

Chapter 4

As time goes by …

Music psychotherapy and trauma

Julie Sutton

Trauma

In the 1942 film *Casablanca*, café-owner Rick Blaine cannot bear to remember as his house pianist and friend Sam sings, "no matter what the future brings, as time goes by," having begun, "you must remember this." This is a moment where what he hears takes Rick back in time to an unbearable place in a past he cannot mourn, reminding us how time has a central place in trauma.

Definitions of trauma have evolved over time (Tutté, 2004) and continue to develop in response to research and society. The term trauma relates to shock, experienced as a catastrophic disruption to our status quo (Bisson, Roberts & Macho, 2003; Caruth, 2014). It is unpredictable, sudden, and from this point on, the world and one's sense of oneself in the world changes forever. With traumatic material, the content reverts to a form of primary process thinking (Sutton & McDougall, 2010; Williams, 2010). Time and space collapse, leaving fragments of experience, where past, present, and future appear simultaneously, alongside the unbearable trauma with which they are fused. It is a visceral, overwhelming experience, felt primarily bodily.

Freud (1923, p. 26) noted how the bodily ego, "is ultimately derived from bodily sensations, chiefly from those springing from the surface of the body." Thus, the ego[1] comprises symbolic representations and meanings stemming from sensations in the body. Freud (ibid.) recognised the fundamental relationship we have with our bodies from the beginning of life, and how we build on this once we gather the capacity for language and move out into the world. We also experience our bodies in time. Freud thought memory related to childhood affects our everyday lives, in the sense of having an ever-present past, reworked in the present (Freud, 1899, 1914, 1916). The potential for the past to impinge in the present, presents a challenge for locating ourselves in time. Our experiences change with our perceptions altering over time, taking on intensely personal overtones (in recalling events we often remember our feelings about them). Green (2009) noted access to psychic material outside time is important, with dream work being a link to what is not within our conscious grasp, and where experience can find form within fluidity of past and present.

The approach: the improvisational music psychotherapy method

Research shows how early the auditory channel is formed and made use of, with locating oneself in time being sound-related from the beginning of life (Fox, 2000; Hannon & Trehub, 2005; Hyde, et al., 2009; Patel, 2010; Strickland, 2002; Trimble & Hesdorffer, 2017). Music is a bodily experience, which we hear in patients' musical improvisations, via an understanding of music as a verb rather than a noun (Small, 1998). This incorporates ideas about improvisation as lived human experience (Sutton, in press). If music is undertaken by people (a verb), rather than studied or consumed (a noun), it becomes a means by which one directly expresses oneself through action. While improvisation is a complex term defying a single interpretation, it is also part of life, occurring in any creative activity and in everyday spontaneous conversation (Sutton, 2018).

As Ratte (1997) noted, improvisation puts us in touch with our bodily ego and our presence at that level. Connecting to and with bodily experiences is the basis for thinking and ultimately a means of finding meaning in our existence (Ferenczi, 1913, 1956). Music psychotherapy improvisations offer patients opportunities to experience and make discoveries about themselves and others from the bodily level. Like free associating, patients are offered space to play as they are able, and to respond to what they hear and experience. I suggest patients choose instruments for us both, with a reflective space after playing where they speak about what is in their mind. These improvisations enable us to hear and experience the patient's mind in their present, as it is linked, enmeshed, or confused with the past. We discover how music is an art of time, in an area between the conscious and unconscious, poised in a space located in and between time present and time past.

Music as an art of time

We can experience time in terms of bodily tensions relating to inner states. These ebb and flow continually with a rhythm of their own, dependent on our overall mood and what impinges from the external world. Developmentally we slowly gather the capacity to put words onto these experiences, which to some extent both contains and communicates them. The origin of this capacity begins in infancy (Stern, 1985; Trevarthen, 2011; Winnicott, 1971), where our first year of life is mainly a non-verbal existence, when we begin to form relationships, alongside which we access language (Klein, 1921/1998; Freud, 1972; Bowlby, 1988; Fonagy, Gergely, Junst, & Target, 2002).

Research shows how musical this first period of life is, during a time when we lay down our relational template. Via a dance of attunement between mother and infant, the infant comes to be aware of affect states, and we can "be with" others throughout life in these ways (Stern, 1985, p. 157). One of Stern's observations centred on the musical timing, placing, and qualities of sound, movement, and touch passing between mother and infant. This continuing process was investigated via detailed video analysis of mothers and babies, showing the delicacy of our first dance (Trevarthen, 1977, 1979), with babies' facility for learning via vocalising and gesturing, through their own effort, revealing matching responses and expressions, as well as awareness of the emotional exchange itself (Trevarthen, 2011). Mothers send out stimuli that have a communicative intent, sometimes pausing and waiting for baby, opening up a space enabling potential digesting of what has occurred at a perceptual bodily level, as well as giving a break from intense activity for both. This is a template for verbal conversation, offered as an experience of relationship (Bion, 2007) and is not mimicry as in copying, but with intent to provide links between both parties in the duet, as a process of attunement.

Music psychotherapists understand how these form-giving experiences are tangible when improvising musically, having detailed awareness of early, relational musical components. These earliest experiences of ourselves take place within an evolving bodily process of emotional connection to others, during which we both reach out and take in experiences, of ourselves and of others. These are musical experiences, as noted by Noy (1968, p. 65), with our strong, immediate response to music related to this early communicative, interactive template. We feel most profoundly music's physical effect and the deeply meaningful experience this brings us on different levels, which is why music is such a powerful and subtle medium in the treatment of those traumatised.

We can be caught between subjective and chronological time, drawn towards the former over the latter. Psychoanalysts broadly agree that we connect with the timelessness of the unconscious and its mental contents via dreaming. When a dream is described in the consulting room it becomes temporal in an everyday sense as the dream is given a narrative that flows in time. In speaking, the dreamer moves into an area between time and timelessness. As Parsons put it, "to tell a dream in the analytic situation is more than narration. It is to expose one's dreaming, and this is to place oneself where time and timelessness collide" (Parsons, 2009, p. 38).

Dreaming is also possible because of the psychotherapist's reverie (Ogden, 1997), that is, their own dreaming when they are with the patient, whether they are improvising or listening with a musically attuned ear (Bion, 2005). Situated in the area between time and timelessness, music where linear temporal reality collides with the atemporality of a timeless, formless or fragmented emptiness can be termed psychotic play, heard via sounded dreams that destroy rather than create time. As music is an art of time, as well as being a means of studying time as it unfolds, the psychotherapist's musical stance in the clinic room makes it possible for patients to have a potential experience of being-in-time, however fleetingly. This emerges through the way psychotherapists listen to the timelessness of the patient's music as it occurs, as in the following example, where repetition halted the possibility of a patient's going-on-being (Winnicott, 1960).

Timeless time: the grey dream

Trauma disrupts our sense of going-on-in-time. Traumatic repetition results from our unsuccessful attempts to manage the impact of traumatic events. Experiences, impressions, and memories are not remembered, but repeatedly experienced, as with flashbacks. This is a stuck, fixed re-experiencing, unless a further, developing phase occurs, where the experiences, impressions, and memories are reactivated, and out of which emerges new meaning (Freud's "Nachträgligkeit"). For some there are traumatic developmental factors as well as experiences of single or multiple traumatic events, such as in war zones (Lord Alderdice, 2017; Sutton, 2002).

In psychotic time, there is no space for anything other than the re-experiencing of traumata, heard in the music of those traumatised. This takes many forms, common to all being characteristics of endlessness (no beginning and no ending), timelessness (no movement forwards or back), shapelessness or formlessness (no phrasing, no development of material), and fragmentation (no sense of continuity). We cannot make sense of this music, just as our patients cannot make sense of what they have experienced. When the traumatised individual plays, we hear repetition without meaning, but we know immediately when this changes, and music 'becomes' in a creative way. This is a different kind of repetition, with space, shape, and an embodied sense of going-on-being in the world. Time is now alive, and we can remember in a way we cannot in traumatic music. We might describe this difference as between melancholic music and music where mourning might take place, where the future is brought to us via our letting go what has past. Traumatic play denies this, having a protective function for the patient for whom loss feels unbearable, as in the film *Casablanca* when Rick insists Sam stops playing, and this first example:

> Jill[2] presented with a history of depression and thoughts of self-harm. In an early session, she chose a piano solo, playing the keys where her fingers fell, with little response to the sounds she made. Her music was repetitive, shapeless and with no sense of time moving forward. Alongside the mechanical nature of random sounds produced, there was a tension in the quality of the harmony created by the clusters of notes played. The mood darkened and brief silences occasionally appeared, where Jill's hands lifted up and shifted position over the piano keys.
>
> More and more piano notes filled the room and space contracted. It became difficult to listen and while I could not make sense of Jill's music, I experienced a strong, at times urgent, desire to understand it. I sensed an increase in tension and slowly this motionless music began to shift towards something that might be shaped in the future, although this had not yet happened. I noted: Jill's music is characterised by fragments of motifs, that seem to be trying to move onwards, but the impression is of endlessness with no continuity. Brief, powerfully empty silences occur, like vacant

spaces contrasting with the endless piano sounds. The silences have no sense of ongoing time. Both the silences and the sounds do not have the kind of meaning that can touch us when we feel moved by music's natural dance of tension and relaxation. This music is at the sensory level, in tension without resolution.

After a quiet period to reflect, Jill spoke of the pain and torment of this tension in these words, "it is like being on a hamster wheel, the hamster wants to get off but cannot, all they can do is hope that someone will open the cage for them." Her words described not only the awfulness of feeling trapped in the traumatic experience, in a place where time was destroyed, but also expressed the transference, mirroring my sense of an unspoken call for rescue (Sandler, 1976). It is reminiscent of an experience Bion had during the First World War, of which he wrote: "The dream was grey, shapeless; horror and dread gripped me. I could not cry out, just as now, many years later, I can find no words." (Bion, 1982, p. 237). As with Jill's music, Bion's dream was timeless, comprising wordless bodily experiences. Remaining present with this timelessness encountered its reality, offering Jill a different experience of being heard. There could then be potential for something new to emerge, as in the next example.

A musical process from timelessness to temporality: from chaos to song

At the time of referral Jerry was eight years old with such a severe non-fluency he almost stopped speaking. Moved from mainstream education to a specialist unit he was finding difficulty containing his feelings. His first sessions were full of energy. He played all the percussion instruments available in a way that was both continuous and fragmented, filling the room with sound. His music was extremely loud, with a heightened sense of pressure and urgency. It is difficult to capture the volume of the activity, but I felt at times that I clung to piano notes as if on the edge of a cliff. Jerry also tested the safety and security of the room, for example climbing onto the window frame or throwing his beaters against the wall, which often whizzed past me en route. Seeing the room afterwards, a staff member commented it was "as if a bomb had hit it." Jerry said nothing during these sessions.

A period of structured, controlled music making followed, where Jerry took the lead, assigning me a role of not knowing. He organised the instruments, indicating by gesture how and when they could be played. This music was mechanical, somewhat contrived, strictly controlled, repetitive and more timeless than the earlier fragmented playing. Without knowing why, I sensed it was important to stay with this. One day Jerry began to whisper inaudibly and from this point things changed.

His voice gaining in strength during the next sessions, Jerry began improvising narratives describing scenes and then scenarios about bombs, being frightened, and not being able to run away because he was hurt. Rather than all sounds being controlled, there was a flow and gathering tempo in his voice. I was now free to play in a way that followed Jerry's narrative, as if painting in sound the pictures he was making with his words. This was improvisation, where shapes and meanings were constructed in time. Jerry's scenarios became stories. Gradually the stories became short plays, in which he took on a range of roles, eventually moving between two characters. Representing these characters at the piano, I responded to the mood, contour, placing, and timbre of his voice, playing either harsh, dissonant music, or plaintive, hurt, and sad music. One improvisation of over an hour developed, where the two characters were in conflict, one punitive and the other terrified, screaming, and protesting. Eventually one seemed to resolve an issue with the other. The tension slowly relaxed and after a period of settling Jerry calmly left the room.

Jerry's psychotherapy drew to a close some months after these intense sessions. His behaviour had settled considerably around the unit. He was communicating confidently verbally with no sign of non-fluency. During his last sessions, he improvised songs about relationships, no longer being lonely, having friends, and feeling happier again. He soon returned to mainstream education. Only after his psychotherapy finished it emerged his father had been working on the day of the Enniskillen bomb,[3] a month prior to Jerry's first session. Jerry's father had not been hurt, but did not return home immediately that day due to the aftermath of the event, because he was a member of a security force. His occupation was not public knowledge. At this point in history, members of the military, police, and prison officers were intimidated by paramilitary groups and, along with anyone working for such organisations, targets for being killed. Understandably, families protected their children during this period, with strategies such as denial and minimising the severity of the situation. Many did not discuss what was happening, leading to a powerful collective mechanism. As an Accident and Emergency consultant during this period described, "People are not just individuals, we are persons, and we are persons in a community. We become what we are within the community. This can powerfully affect our feelings, our perceptions and our behaviour, and often we are unaware of this." (Rutherford in Smyth & Fay, 2000, p. 97). Collective and individual silence became a fundamental aspect of managing what was happening in one's community. Literature appearing after the Good Friday Agreement in 1998 bears this out, when many people began speaking for the first time about their experiences (as in the above example, see p. 000). These collective responses reverted to an either-or split, with few individuals providing a third perspective (Dunne, 1995, p. 11).

Within the context of his environment, Jerry's story was uniquely his. The silence at home, in the community and in society was echoed in his silence. As with society, Jerry kept in what could not be allowed to flow out, including terrible, unthinkable anxieties, that can be as Green noted, "terrifying and, ultimately unrepresentable" (Green, 2002, p. 110). Thus we connect the destructive strands and layers of trauma, locating them in a single, complex moment in time, affecting the individual via their personal history, their family, society, the environment, and the influence of the past at all these levels. It is this intersection of factors that is characteristic of the trauma experienced by those living in areas of conflict, where not only thought, but time itself has to be held back. Jerry had to know it was safe to make sounds to be heard, however powerful, fragmented, chaotic, and incomprehensible they were. What emerged initially was explosive, like a psychic bomb exploding, linked to a real bomb, given shape in his later improvised story, beginning, "one day a big bomb came; this was the sound of it." Psychotherapy became a space where we made time for Jerry in a way that built up a continuity of experience. Rather than visiting a community in conflict, working then leaving again, I was also a member of his community, providing another, tangible sense of continuity.

The final example returns to Jill, offering a detailed exploration of a shift, when temporal and atemporal time can be in flux. Potential flow towards a future is then possible, even for those who have had to destroy time because of profoundly traumatic life experiences.

Temporal and atemporal time in flux: repetition in creative time

Jill is now six months further on in her music psychotherapy. She sits opposite me at the metallaphone, choosing it without thinking, apart from previous positive experiences when I accompanied at the piano. Today she wants me to play the same instrument she does. She picks up two beaters, handing one to me.

> Jill begins by playing a single note, after which she hesitates. Prepared to listen but not necessarily play, I sense another note could be possible, and play quietly. During this time, Jill has lifted her beater. Now she plays again, followed a little later by another note from me. This pattern continues, with single notes occurring in turn (Jill-me-Jill-me etc.). From uncertain beginnings, a regularity to the turn taking appears. I experience this as mechanical, functional and more like a metronome marking time. As in her piano solo, rather than all of her, only Jill's arms play her music.
>
> Then, out of nowhere, something else happens: a possible pulse, a kind of heartbeat underlying the music. I sense a different kind of time is possible and that I can play a sound after Jill's, which momentarily creates a pulse. It is like an in-breath before singing, or leaning towards the first step in a dance (Alvarez, 2012, pp. 56–57). There is then a different pattern, as if an interrupted heartbeat: Jill-me ... Jill-me ... Jill-me. While still mechanical, sometimes there is also a leaning towards something alive and "in movement," as of a shape beginning to be formed.

This occurs more often and a different mood emerges. I feel something is happening. It is impossible to know what this is; it is intangible, but present. My notes recorded how, completely unexpectedly, the music felt alive: "While we still exchange single notes in turn, now it sounds like one person playing. The music has a clear dynamic and direction. It has a shape and a form. There are accents marking the beginning and ends of phrases. There is a rise and fall in dynamic and timbre that follows this contour. The music moves forward and dances, with a freedom and space in the phrases being formed. Neither Jill nor I know how this is happening, yet it feels inevitable. We do not know what note to play, but when played, it is the note that should be played. We follow the music as if it is playing us. The exchange between us has speeded up. We both seem to be in flow, dancing the sticks onto the instrument. Jill looks up for the first time, surprised, excited, and smiling.

After a while this music reaches the end of a phrase and then collapses. I feel lost, and there is a return to the previous mechanical turn-taking. Sooner than before, the same things emerge and there is another period of lively, alive music, again as if one person is playing. After a silence this stops, and Jill says, "something happened, something new I never felt before."

This example demonstrates the beginning or initial stages of what Green (2002) called a capacity for enduring; how a bodily attuning presence can provide an environmental difference (a presence around the patient), contributing to Jill's new experience of herself. Green wrote, "Who can deny that the intervention of the object, simply by its presence, can help to transform the situation dominated by suffering and frustration, thereby favouring the transition to secondary process and elaboration" (Green, 2002, p. 119). In music psychotherapy, this kind of presence is made possible by the quality and temporality of the therapist's musical identity (their embodied musicianship, developed across time) alongside their therapeutic identity (training, personal psychotherapy, lifelong learning).

When repetition has a subjective relationship to the past, the painful process of mourning can be borne, so the future becomes possible. In this new space we find restorative, reparative processes. A new music emerges, within which the psychotherapist's musical stance is central, incorporating an ability to stay with timelessness (both temporal and atemporal). A facility with utilising a musical identity and flexibility with different ways of listening and playing in the clinic room go alongside this, as well as listening from a deep, layered awareness of what is sounded, both in sound and silence. When society destroys time as in armed conflict and war, we have further layers of experience that have potential to be viewed differently via the passage of time. As we know, the Northern Ireland peace process has not resulted in peace inside the people most affected. In societies where anxiety can be at psychotic levels, there is compulsion to feel in control but no room for difference. This may be why there can continue to be a powerful and sometimes seductive draw to the past, as if time itself can be made to stand still. Jill and Jerry were from such a context, with further complexity where early nurturing environments were impinged upon by external events encompassing unpredictable violence, the nature of which changed over time.

The construction of reality: as time goes by

I have aimed to cover experiences of different aspects of time in the clinic room to orientate the reader to core qualities of music. Improvisation is a means of self-construction, making time for oneself and for others. Thinking about phenomena in the clinic room from musical and analytical theoretical perspectives opens up spaces for understanding the complicated layers and contexts trauma presents. While repetition in earlier life is a bedrock from which growth occurs, we can understand developmental and environmental trauma as an experience of shock and overwhelm, occurring in recurrent patterns that affect attachment and development as a whole, particularly sensitising the individual to later similar repetitions (Bigda-Peyton, 2000; Castillo & Bailey, 2002; Lynch, 2000). As trauma destroys time, it is through mourning that we have a truly temporal existence, with its potential for the painful, reparative processing of loss. Music perhaps above all the arts, allows opportunities for this, because it is both an art of time and an embodied experience (De Backer & Sutton, 2014). The musical medium also requires delicate handling when working with those traumatised as it can so easily overwhelm.

With musical qualities of presence, strands of experiences might exist as if they were individual lines of polyphonic musical textures, but with the score written in time, via improvisation. Psychoanalysts interested in music have also noticed aspects of these ideas. Segal provided clues relating to the power the arts have in offering creative time travel, stating how, "for the artist, the work of art is his most complete and satisfactory way of allaying the guilt and despair arising out of the depressive position and of restoring his destroyed objects" (Segal, 1952, p. 198). Sabbadini thought that analytic work might proceed, "As if we were musicians, [where] we help our analysands to enrich with sounds the frightening silence of the void they carry inside." (Sabbadini, 2014, p. 140). Harris Williams went further, noting how, "in psychoanalysis, the verbal "talking cure" and the visual nature of dreams have overshadowed its musical resonances. If we learn to observe and appreciate this hidden music, we will become better symbol-makers and less reliant on sign systems" (Harris Williams, 2010, p. 157).

In these ways, awareness of the musical, fluctuating qualities of temporality and atemporality addresses fundamental aspects of trauma: of past, present and future, of before, and after. This facilitates emerging potential spaces for remembering what we were, and as we do this, to move towards what we have yet to become, as time goes by.

Notes

1 Ego: what we mean when we use the term "I."
2 The names of patients have been changed to protect their privacy.
3 A bomb went off during a Remembrance Day ceremony at Enniskillen War Memorial in 1987. 11 people died including 3 married couples and 13 children. Over 60 were injured. It was one of the first times amateur film footage was broadcast.

References

Alvarez, A. (2012). *The thinking heart. Three levels of psychoanalytic therapy with disturbed children*. Hove/New York: Routledge.

Bigda-Peyton, F. (2000). An analysis of intense enactments in the case of a 10-year-old girl. *Mod. Psychoanalysis*, 25(2), 227–248.

Bion, W. R. (1982/2005). *The long week-end 1879–1919. Part of a life*. London/New York: Karnac.

Bion, W. R. (2005). *The Tavistock seminars*. Edited by F. Bion. London/New York: Karnac.

Bion, W. R. (2007). *Second thoughts*. London/New York: Karnac. (first published in 1967).

Bisson, J. I., Roberts, N., & Macho, G. (2003). The Cardiff traumatic stress initiative: An evidence-based approach to early psychological intervention following traumatic events. *Psychiatric Bulletin*, 27, 145–147.

Bowlby, J. (1988). *A secure base: Clinical applications of attachment theory*. London: Hogarth Press & Institute of Psychoanalysis.

Caruth, C. (2014). Book review. Lost in transmission: Studies of trauma across generations edited by M. Gerard Fromm. Karnac, London2012. *International Journal of Psychoanalysis* 95(2), 402–407.

Castillo, A., Bailey, J. (2002). Holding and treating the traumatized child: A preschooler's resilience in mastering his fears and making sense of his life. *Infant Child Adolescent Psychotherapy*, 2(1), 67–93.

De Backer, J. & Sutton, J. (2014). (Eds.) *The music in music therapy. Psychodynamic music therapy in Europe: Clinical, theoretical and research perspectives*. London /Philadelphia: Jessica Kingsley.

Dunne, S. (1995). (Ed.) *Facets of the conflict in Northern Ireland*. Hampshire/London: MacMillan Press.

Ferenczi, S. (1913/1956). *Stages in the development of the sense of reality. Sex in psychoanalysis*. New York: Dover Publications.

Fonagy, P., Gergely, G., Jurist, E. L., & Target, M. (2002). *Affect regulation, mentalization, and the development of the self*. New York: Other Books.

Fox, D. B. (2000). Music and the baby's brain. *Music Educators Journal*, 87(2), 23–29.

Freud, A. (1972). The child as a person in his own right. *Psychoanalytic Study of The Child* 27, 621–625.

Freud, S. (1899). Screen memories. S.E., Vol. 3. (pp. 301–322). London: Hogarth.

Freud, S. (1914). Remembering, repeating and working-through. S.E., Vol. 12 (pp. 145–156). London: Hogarth.

Freud, S. (1916). On transience. S.E., Vol. 14 (pp. 303–308). J. Strachey, Ed. London: Hogarth.

Freud, S. (1923). S.E., Vol. 19. London: Hogarth.

Green, A. (2002). *Time in psychoanalysis. Some contradictory aspects*. London/New York: Free Association Books.

Green, A. (2009). From the ignorance of time to the murder of time. From the murder of time to the misrecognition of temporality on psychoanalysis. In L. G. Fiorini, J. Canestri (Eds.), *The Experience of Time. Psychoanalytic Perspectives* (pp. 1–19). London: Karnac.

Hannon, E. E. & Trehub, S. E. (2005). Tuning in to musical rhythms: Infants learn more readily than adults. *Proceedings of the National Academy of Sciences of the United States of America*, 102(35), 12639–12643.

Harris Williams, M. (2010). *The aesthetic development. The poetic spirit of psychoanalysis*. London & New York: Karnac.

Hyde, K. L., Lerch, J., Norton, A., Forgeard, M., Winner, E., & Evans, A. C. (2009). Musical training shapes structural brain development. *The Journal of Neuroscience*, 29, 3019–3025.

Klein, M. (1921/1998). The development of a child. In *Love, guilt and reparation & other works 1921–1945* (pp. 1–53). USA: The Free Press & The Melanie Klein Trust.

Lord Alderdice, J. (2017). Fundamentalism, radicalization and terrorism. Part 2: Fundamentalism, regression and repair. *Psychoanalytic Psychotherapy*, 31(3), 301–313.

Lynch, M. (2000). The role of the body as the medium in child psychotherapy: Snapshots of therapy with an 11-year-old, severely abused, multiply placed girl. *Journal of Child Psychotherapy* 26 (2), 159–181.

Noy, P. (1968). The development of musical ability. *The Psychoanalytical Study of the Child*, 23, 332–347.

Ogden, T. (1997). *Reverie and interpretation. Sensing something human*. New Jersey: Jason Aronson.

Parsons, M. (2009). Why did Orpheus look back? In L. G. Fiorini & J. Canestri (Eds.), *The Experience of time. Psychoanalytic perspectives* (pp. 35–43). London: Karnac.

Patel, A. D. (2010). Music, biological evolution, and the brain. *Emerging Disciplines*, 91–144.

Ratte, M. (1997). Improvisation as form. *Resonance*, 6(1).

Sabbadini, A. (2014). *Boundaries and bridges. Perspectives on time and space in psychoanalysis*. London/New York: Karnac.

Sandler, J. (1976). Countertransference and role-responsiveness. *International Journal of Psychoanalysis*, 3, 43–47.

Segal, H. (1952). A psycho-analytical approach to aesthetics. *International Journal of Psychoanalysis*, 33, 196–207.

Small, C. (1998). *Musicking. The meanings of performing and listening*. Middletown, CT: Wesleyan University Press.

Smyth, M. & Fay, M-T. (2000). (Eds.) *William Rutherford interview: All in a day's work. Personal accounts from Northern Ireland's troubles.* (pp. 96–102). London & Sterling, Virginia: Pluto Press.

Stern, D. (1985). *The interpersonal world of the infant*. New York: Basic Books.

Strickland, S. J. (2002). Music and the brain in childhood development. *Childhood Education*, 78(2), 100–103.

Sutton, J. (2018). "The invisible handshake": A backdrop for improvisation in music therapy. *British Journal of Music Therapy*, 32(2), 86–95.

Sutton, J. (in press) Fresh, uncut, uncensored: Exploring the intersubjective dimensions of improvisation. *Contemporary Music Review*.

Sutton, J. & McDougall, I. (2010). The roar on the other side of silence: Some thoughts about silence and the traumatic in music therapy. In K. Stewart (Ed.), *Music therapy & trauma. Bridging theory and clinical practice* (pp. 88–100). New York: Satchmo Press.

Sutton, J. P. (2002). (Ed.) *Music, music therapy and trauma. International perspectives.* London/Philadelphia: Jessica Kingsley.

Trevarthen, C. (1977). Descriptive analyses of infant communicate behaviour. In H. R. Shaffer (Ed.), *Studies in mother-infant interaction.* (pp. 227–270). New York: Academic Press.

Trevarthen, C. (1979). Communication and cooperation in early infancy: A description of primary intersubjectivity. In M. M. Bullow (Ed.) *Before speech: The beginning of interpersonal communication* (pp. 231–348). New York: Cambridge University Press.

Trevarthen, C. (2011). What is it like to be a person who knows nothing? Defining the active intersubjective mind of a newborn human being. *Infant and Child Development*, 20(1), 119–135.

Trimble, M., Hesdorffer, D. (2017). Music and the brain: The neuroscience of music and musical appreciation. *British Journal of Psychiatry Int.*, 14(2), 28–31.

Tutté, J.C. (2004). The concept of psychical trauma: A bridge in interdisciplinary space. *International Journal of Psycho-Analysis*, 85(4), 897–921.

Williams, P. (2010). *Invasive objects. Minds under siege.* New York/London: Routledge/Taylor & Francis.

Winnicott, D. W. (1960). The theory of the parent-infant relationship. *International Journal of Psychoanalysis*, 41, 585–595.

Winnicott, D. W. (1971). *Playing and reality.* Tavistock, UK: Tavistock Publications.

Chapter 5

Healing trauma through embodied relating

Re-establishing rhythms of relating

Gill Westland

Introduction

Vera is a composite client and the author's work with her illustrates the theory described in this chapter. This chapter discusses impaired movement patterns and how in unresolved trauma these affect relationships. It focuses on work with adults who have experienced early developmental trauma.

> Vera is in her early 30s and describes her mother as "borderline." She was fine one moment, then she would lash out in a rage about something minor and nothing would console her. Vera's mother was orphaned at an early age and grew up in a children's home. Vera's father was a "violent alcoholic." When sober he was "nasty" and Vera has had no contact with him for years. Vera is intelligent, a "survivor" who has a partner and demanding work in a care agency. She is good at thinking on her feet and solving problems. However, her attitudes are inflexible; she "overthinks" continuously, finds it hard to rest and sleep in spite of tiredness. She is often exhausted by her heroic efforts to deal with the many things that she feels are her responsibility. Apart from herself, she trusts no one to do anything properly. She learned at an early age to look after herself and this was exacerbated when, at the age of seven years, her aunt died. Time spent infrequently with her aunt had given her some respite from the danger of her family home. Then it was gone.

The body provides the capacity to survive and resolve traumatic experiences, but trauma affects the body and any unprocessed traumatic experiences are encoded in the body (van der Kolk, 1994). Trauma involves life-threatening events as well as those *perceived* as life threatening. "All trauma is preverbal" (van der Kolk, 2014, p. 43) as it affects the body, although the individual may not be conscious of its effects on their behaviour and emotions. Nevertheless, the remnants of traumatic experiences are recognisable in diminished and strange body sensations, restricted breathing, and limited range of movements. The restrictions of movements are within recognised norms and not attributable to any physical injury or impairment. Frequently, emotional expression is stunted or flooding, or a mixture of the two extremes as the traumatised person is unable to manage their feelings and the accompanying physiological processes. The impact of traumatic events is often multi-layered, chained together, and difficult to disentangle. These are a mixture of survival, intergenerational, epigenetic, and traumatic attachment phenomena.

> As Vera related events from her life in general and her childhood during the first consultation, it seemed likely that she carried different sorts of traumatic experiences. Vera's way of being was congruent with this. Her body barely moved as she spoke, and when asked about her body sensations, she described numb legs and being hot and cold in different parts of her body. She knew that her childhood was traumatic, but her efforts to resolve it through online resources and books had not helped much.
>
> The complex and physical nature of trauma often makes it inaccessible to therapeutic modalities, which rely on the spoken word and lack the somatic dimension. Thus a bodily based approach, which concentrates on body sensations and movements, is the main route for processing trauma (see for example, Ogden, Minton, & Pain, 2006; Rothschild, 2000, 2017). This offers a direct way of resolving traumatic experiences privileging the non-verbal dimensions of relating, but not excluding verbal communication. Vera's difficulties called for a bodily based approach.

During early babyhood, repeated, mostly non-verbal, interactions between babies and carers become physically embedded. These interactions involve carers recognising their baby's communications, noticing when their baby cannot soothe or stimulate (self-regulate) themselves and giving help when needed (interactive regulating) (Beebe & Lachmann, 2002). The baby-carer interactions flow like a "dance," sometimes the baby leading, sometimes the carer, and sometimes both "dancing together" (Brazelton, Koslowski, & Main, 1974). Movements and regulation go hand in hand. The carer knows, for example, when to slow their movements down, back away a bit, and soften their voice to give the baby space to follow their drowsiness. Psychotherapy with traumatised people involves finding the "dance" that did not develop in babyhood. The therapeutic task is to tune into the client's movement patterns, to support the client's awareness of them, and find new movements. Indeed, "psychotherapy can be seen as a means of restoring coherent, integrated movement on multiple levels" (Caldwell, 2017, p. 54).

Developmental trauma and movement

Developmental trauma arises from the lack of predictable safety in insecure attachment relationships. When babies feel safe and loved, they feel secure, and without this consistently they feel insecure. Of note is that insecure disorganised/traumatic attachment (Main and Solomon, 1986) is linked with later borderline personality disorder, post-traumatic stress disorder, and dissociation (Beebe, Lachmann, Markese, & Bahrick, 2012; Beebe, Lachmann, Markese, Buck, et al., 2012; Schore, 2003). Carers within insecure disorganised attachments relate erratically, are intrusive and aggressive, often interfering and menacing in so-called "play" and, at the other extreme, absent or distant (Hesse & Main, 1999). *Vera's babyhood suggested an insecure disorganised attachment with her mother.*

Early ways of relating are physically felt by babies. Sensing one's own feelings, and the intentions of others and their feelings involves muscle movement (Porges, 2011). This is so fundamental that newborns have the capacity to move in time with their adult caregivers (Trevarthen, 2009). In traumatised attachments, babies diminish their movements in self protection, but at the cost of relating fully. The first fifteen months is significant for the development of the right brain and communication is mostly non-verbal (Schore, 1994). The right brain modulates emotional arousal, regulates stress, takes in whole situations, and is important in empathy, creativity, humour, intuition, and non-verbal communication (McGilchrist, 2009). Where carers are more attuned than not, the carer magnifies positive emotional states and diminishes negative ones. Movement, breathing, and regulation are well harmonised and the right brain develops well enough. The insecurely attached baby in contrast has irregular rhythms of relating with movement, breathing, and regulation being impaired. Whether secure or insecure, the oft repeated baby-carer interactions establish *signature patterns of relating*, which are revealed in *signature patterns of moving* (Westland, 2015). These relational patterns have familiar movements, rhythms, pace, emotional intensity, and so on, and are expressive of feelings. Movements change according to how someone is feeling and what the person wants to express in a context. Adult clients reveal their signature patterns of relating in gestures, movement or lack of it (e.g. arms hanging limply, talking with little movement in the chest), breathing style, modes of emotional expression (excessive or limited), capacity to think and so on. *In the early stages with Vera, she was fiercely "right" in the disputes she recounted; she had very limited space for another point of view. Her immobile and taut body reflected this.*

Movements and stress in the embryo

Attachment trauma may be blended with intergenerational stress. Bowers and Yehuda (2016), for example, argue that stress can be transmitted by parents through gametes, the uterine environment, as well as care after birth. The effects of stress are reflected in neuroendocrine, epigenetic, and neuroanatomy changes. The embryologist, Blechschmidt describes developmental movements in the embryo and foetus generated by directional forces, which are essential for optimum development (Blechschmidt, 1977). He argues that even minor disturbances in the movements of the metabolic processes at this stage of development have enormous impact incrementally on the potential development of the embryo, causing "malfunctions" (Blechschmidt, 1977, p. 7) and sometimes even death. The malfunctions may be within normal limits, but set up a trajectory of development. They influence the potential for resilience or vulnerability. The minor disturbances may be from drugs, infections, substances, which are not noxious in other circumstances, hereditary disease, and "bad shock" (Blechscmidt, 1977, p. 99).

Signature patterns of movement

A clinically useful model for thinking about signature movement patterns is that of *motoric fields* (Boadella, 2000a; Boadella, 2000b). These are paired and contrasted movement patterns. Boadella draws on Blechschmidt (1977), Laban's movement analysis, (Laban & Lawrence, 1974) and Janet's work on movement attitude, movement memory, and motoric self (Janet, 1929, cited in Boadella, 2000a), for his elaboration of motoric fields. In trauma, the free flow of movement between each pole of a movement is a possibility, but is usually impaired in some way (Boadella, 2000a; Boadella, 2000b). The different motoric fields represent an individual's capacity for relating in different spheres.

The motoric fields (Boadella, 2000a; Boadella, 2000b) are Absorption and Activation, Flexion and Extension, Traction and Opposition, and Rotation and Canalisation. Absorption involves relative stillness for recuperation and taking in. Activation is the impulse to move, to express oneself, and make contact with others. Depressed clients get stuck in absorption without being nourished by the inactivity and find it difficult to get moving. Activation for many individuals is tense and driven rather than pleasurable. It is the pattern of the workaholic seeking approval through effort but gaining no satisfaction. In Flexion muscles bend towards the body. Extension is the opposite movement away from the body. Emotionally flexion of both arms expresses "come closer to me" and extension with the palms facing outwards expresses "that's far enough, give me some space" (see, for example, Marcher & Fich, 2010). Traction involves pulling and Opposition involves pushing with some sustained force. Combining Traction (pulling) with Flexion of the arms involves pulling someone or something towards us. Pushing (Opposition) involves creating personal boundaries and preventing invasion. Rotation is going towards something indirectly and is meandering. Canalisation is focused and direct. Someone can walk purposefully to a venue, or go on a country walk following whims. The integration of all of these movement styles is Pulsation. Pulsation involves expanding out into the environment, followed by moving inwards. It represents reaching for contact with others and expressing oneself, and then being with oneself to recharge without feeling lonely. Free flowing pulsation has a regular rhythm to it. Generally, the less pulsation is inhibited, the more easy and flexible are relationships with oneself and others and the more alive someone feels. *Vera exhibited restrictions in each of these motoric fields at the beginning of psychotherapy.*

Unrealised potential

Signature patterns of movement contain both trauma-related dynamics and "unrealised potential" or "essence" (Southwell, 2010, p. 11). Other terms used for this latent potential are "core" (Lowen, 1973, p. 312) and "essential Self" (Rosenberg, Rand, & Asay, 1985, p. 23). Traumatised individuals, therefore, always have the possibility of developing "unrealised potential" (Boening, Southwell, & Westland, 2012, p. 5).

Boyesen described the "primary personality" (Boyesen, 1976, p. 81) for someone living life from their core. This carries spiritual connotations as well as biological ones. Primary impulse(s) and primary communications (Westland, 2015) are linked with the primary personality. If our early relationships are harsh or the atmosphere of the home is threatening, primary impulses become overlaid and obscured by secondary ones, which become relatively fixed (Southwell, 1988). The acquired secondary communications (Boadella, 1987; Westland, 2015) with their physical patterns (secondary patterns) represent the way a child protected themselves from experiencing unbearable feelings. The secondary patterning in traumatised adults is revealed in signature patterns of movements with their accompanying dysregulation of physiology and feelings. It obscures the inherent potential. Reminding them of their inherent health is a way to help clients to stabilise themselves in the early stages of psychotherapy. Questions such as "How did you survive that?" and "What helps?" often do this. *For Vera, this was the time spent with her aunt on her farm. Vera's eyes lit up briefly as she recounted playing with Bonzo, her aunt's Labrador. Memories of this kept her going when she was not with her aunt.*

Embodied relating

Trevarthen (2009) supports the use of:

> non-verbal intersubjective therapies such as … body psychotherapy because these approaches accept that we are all equipped with a sensitivity for movement and qualities in movement, not only in our own bodies but in the bodies of others we touch, see and hear.
>
> (Trevarthen, 2009, p. 84)

Central to this is embodied relating, which requires the psychotherapist *living in* a body. This entails physically sensing experiences, and being aware of and *reflecting* on them, whether thinking, feeling, imagining, moving, speaking, and so on. This awareness is moment by moment. Any talking by the psychotherapist, for example, is done with reference to how the words are vibrating in their own body, and monitoring their impact on the client's body through observation. In contrast, *disembodied relating* is *having a body*, and thinking about it without any bodily awareness. Reflecting on bodily experiences is not the same as thinking and mentalising about the body (Sletvold, 2014; Westland, 2015). Awareness gives the possibility of psychotherapist and client being in contact with each other. When contact is there (as when babies and carers are in tune) clients feel seen, met, and understood. They feel recognised as more than their trauma. Contact fosters safety and enables the therapeutic dyad to take risks and explore. The psychotherapist's job is to foster the client's awareness of their body so that they can take charge of themselves. This facilitates the pacing of the session, with self and interactive regulations modulating autonomic nervous system (ANS) processes, emotions, and energy. Focusing on the body with awareness prevents clients being re-traumatised, and vicarious traumatisation and burnout is less likely in psychotherapists (Ogden, Minton, & Pain, 2006; Rothschild, 2000). As clients gain more capacity for independent well-being through improved self-regulation and the establishment of new movement patterns, living with the exhaustion of unresolved trauma is replaced with more vitality.

> After about six months of psychotherapy, Vera is calmer and her movements and speech are slower through improved self regulation. She is less easily triggered into angry reactions with those who had "wronged" her in daily life. She is less critical of me for not being sufficiently on her side. Early on, I intuited, that her vengeful rage (secondary communications) masks the child living in her, who is terrified of her mother and father. This has helped me not to react to her anger towards me. As we have had increasing moments of contact Vera has developed some inner space, can increasingly think about her actions, and explore.
>
> Vera arrives for her session having been catapulted into her usual angry, reactive patterns. Work is being re-organised and her job will be disappearing. She talks quickly about what she is going to do to the management, cranking herself up emotionally and there is no room for any verbal response from me. I listen quietly and calmly and stay embodied until her tirade finishes (self and interactive regulation). I suggest that we might explore her reactions to the work re-organisation by standing and moving. She is open to this. She moves for a while following her inner movements and we arrive at her wanting to explore Pushing (Opposition) together. She pushes against the wall and then against me. If we did not have firm rules in place, she could easily push me across the room. I experience her hands pushing against mine as stiff like steel. There is no contact in her touch. She simply takes her position and pushes. She likes the feeling of power and that she can brush me aside, if she chooses. This is the way to deal with a problem. Her rigid thinking is reflected in her rigid movements. However, Vera ruefully reflects that she gains no lasting satisfaction from this way of going on in the world. Often, she feels that there is no one to help her, so she has no other choice.

We decide to explore her pulling me towards her with her arms (Traction). She feels nothing, and her arms lack force. Vera is puzzled by why she would want to pull someone towards her. We continue to explore pushing and pulling, and moving between the two movements. We end the session with her bafflement about pulling. Without saying anything she seems to know that there is something here to explore further. She leaves quietly and thoughtfully. She has gained some awareness of herself in relationships.

The exploration of Traction and Opposition revealed to Vera a major aspect of her signature patterns of movement.

Rhythms of relating

Hypotoned and hypertoned muscle

Signature patterns of relating are revealed in adults in gross movements, as Vera demonstrates. It is the action of particular muscle groups, which makes movements. In traumatised clients muscles may be over-toned and excessively tense (hypertoned) or limp and without enough tone (hypotoned), or a mixture of under and over-toned muscles (for example, Heller, 2012). Individuals with a preponderance of under-toned muscles will have difficulties with knowing and containing what they feel. These individuals tend to flood, invade, and merge with others. Those with over-toned muscle in quantity tend to be intransigent and distant. At the extremes, those with mixed patterns of under and over-toned muscles can swing between being distant and merging, and be confusing to those around them. *Vera had over-toned arm extensor muscles and under-toned flexor muscles.* The different muscle patterns and their tone can change quickly when a client is reminded of past events. Muscle tone goes hand in hand with physiological and emotional regulation. Early developmental trauma becomes activated in the transference dynamics of the therapeutic relationship. In the activation, clients are unable to regulate emotions and physiology. Over-arousal is linked with the feelings of panic, terror, and rage, and under-arousal with shame, disgust, and despair (Schore, 2009).

Vera's default position was over-arousal and rage. Inevitably in psychotherapy she was dysregulated at times, but the working principle was to let her "reexperience dysregulating affects *in affectively tolerable doses in the context of a safe environment*" (Schore, 2009, p. 130, original italics) and to re-direct the experiences and energy driving the dysregulation.

States of arousal in traumatised clients

Self-regulation and arousal levels in traumatised clients is complex. Brantbjerg (2018) outlines three survival reactions with different levels of arousal requiring

different therapeutic responses: freeze/alert, freeze/fight (which has some readiness to action in it), and immobilisation (under- and over-arousal simultaneously). *Mostly Vera moved between freeze/alert and freeze/fight in sessions.*
   Alongside monitoring movements, Schore states that:

> the psychobiologically attuned empathic therapist, on a moment-to-moment basis, implicitly tracks and matches the patterns of rhythmic crescendos/decrescendos of the patient's regulated and dysregulated ANS with his or her own ANS crescendos/decrescendos. When the patterns of synchronized rhythms are in interpersonal resonance, this right-brain to right-brain specifically fitted interaction generates amplified energetic processes of arousal, and this interactive affect regulation, in turn, cocreates an intersubjective field.
>
> (Schore, 2009, p. 132)

The psychotherapist observes changes in the client's physiology. The client may, for example, turn pale, go still, or their face flush red. Concurrently, the psychotherapist observes themselves and makes adjustments to their level of arousal. They may also direct the client to make adjustments. The psychotherapist's self adjustments will have an impact on the client and is at the heart of self and interaction regulation. *When Vera was venting a torrent of angry words, I breathed out fully, took full in-breaths, and widened my trunk. This served to lower Vera's over-arousal shown in her venting. My actions kept us both less over-aroused. Over time, Vera gradually lowered her arousal without it being spoken about.*
   When focusing on right brain to right brain relating as described by Schore (2009) the task is also to tune into what is unspoken in the client and yet communicated through gesture, tone of voice, movements, breathing patterns (Westland, 2015). Much of this way of relating is intuitive and spontaneous (Marks-Tarlow, 2013).

Additional psychotherapy skills

So far, body awareness, a focus on movements, and the regulation of physiology and emotions have been discussed. Additionally, psychotherapists working with traumatised clients benefit from *monitoring levels of consciousness* in themselves and clients. Levels of consciousness range from "matter of fact," through to "deep emotional" (Westland, 2015, p. 130). The matter of fact level is close to everyday consciousness and is evident in giving information to someone. The deep emotional level is full of feelings towards someone or something. After recognising the level, the psychotherapist makes a choice about how to adjust the level for therapeutic benefit. This might involve, for example, speaking more matter of factly or asking a question requiring a factual response to shift a client from the deep emotional level to the matter of fact level to prevent overwhelm. Monitoring levels of consciousness goes alongside "long rein" and "short rein" holding (Westland, 2015, p. 92). This is like the psychotherapist holding the client on an imaginary lead. Short rein holding keeps the client tightly in the relationship, in present time, without silences and with little room for emotions to surface. Long rein holding leaves the client with more room to explore and potentially deepen into their feelings. Over the course of a session the holding is adjusted to therapeutic need. The moment by moment awareness of these different dimensions of relating and responding to their different rhythms and making adjustments enables new ways of relating to emerge. Making choices about how to go on in this form of psychotherapy is spontaneous and intuitive, rather than goal-directed.

In a later session, Vera illustrates some of this in practice.

> Vera arrives more exhausted than I have ever seen her. She is to lose her job. I suggest that she let herself be exhausted and lie down on the mattress. She nods and lies on her side tightly curled up; she is restless and tries different positions, but is frustrated. She asks me to sit close and curls up on her front with her legs tucked up under her. I place a hand in the middle of her upper back. I intuit that she needs my help to rest and she has contracted for touch to be part of her therapy at the start. Touch can quickly decrease arousal. The atmosphere shifts. After a while, she speaks of her aunt sitting with her at bedtime. Vera's breathing deepens (her arousal is coming down). She turns slightly towards me and her fingers reach for my other hand. She pulls it closer to herself. She cries softly. Later she tells me that she is crying for all the lost life ... she recognises how unkind she has been to the little girl in her.

Unusually, Vera had been able to let herself dwell in Absorption. From this, the movement of Traction emerged (primary impulse). She let herself surrender to feelings of vulnerability, and unusually reached out to another. With this came grief and new vitality. Her job loss had not changed, but her relationship to it had more possibilities. She had shifted from preoccupation with the everyday situation to deepening into the feelings provoked by it. The therapeutic holding was closer to matter of fact at the beginning of the session and moved into deeper emotional holding.

Conclusions

As Vera explored her signature patterns of movements, her range of movements expanded and she and her relationships changed. She became less stubborn about doing things her way. She sought help from others and was surprised when it was offered without her asking. Our relationship became more two way and I was able to offer a different view from Vera's without her flying off the handle. Our interactions became more flowing, and with more give and take in them. We worked throughout with the physicality of her trauma and did not speak about specific traumatic events of her life, apart from naming some of them, but her trauma symptoms lessened. Over time Vera was less in the grip of her past and could make more choices. This could have been the end of psychotherapy. However, Vera wanted more than this and continued with psychotherapy. She illustrates that transformation can happen without being consciously known and spoken about (Lyons-Ruth, 1998).

References

Beebe, B. & Lachmann, F. M. (2002). *Infant research and adult treatment: Co-constructing interactions*. New York: The Analytic Press.

Beebe, B., Lachmann, F. M., Markese, S., & Bahrick, L. (2012). On the origins of disorganised attachment and internal working models: Paper I. A dyadic systems approach. *Psychoanalytic Dialogues: The International Journal of Relational Perspectives*, 22(2), 253–272.

Beebe, B., Lachmann, F. M., Markese, S., Buck, K. A., Bahrick, L., Chen, H., *et al.*, (2012). On the origins of disorganised attachment and internal working models: Paper II. An empirical microanalysis of 4-month mother-infant interaction. *Psychoanalytic Dialogues: The International Journal of Relational Perspectives*, 22(3), 352–374.

Blechschmidt, E. (1977). *The beginnings of human life*. New York: Springer-Verlag.

Boadella, D. (1987). *Lifestreams: An introduction to Biosynthesis*. London: Routledge and Kegan Paul.

Boadella, D. (2000a). Shape flow and postures of the soul. The Biosynthesis concept of the motoric fields. *Energy and Character*, 30(2), 7–17, April2000.

Boadella, D. (2000b). The historical development of the concept of the motoric fields. *Energy and Character*, 30(2), 18–21.

Boening, M., Southwell, C., & Westland, G. (July2012). UK Body Psychotherapy Competencies. www.eabp.org/forum-body-psychotherapy-competencies.php.

Bowers, M. E. & Yehuda, R. (2016). Intergenerational transmission of stress in humans. *Neuropsychopharmacology Reviews*, 41, 232–244.

Boyesen, G. (1976). The primary personality and its relationship to the streamings. In Boadella, D. (Ed.) (1993). *In the wake of Reich* (pp. 81–98). London: Coventure.

Brantbjerg, M.H. (2018). From autonomic reactivity to empathic resonance in psychotherapy mutual regulation of post-traumatic stress (PTS). What does that take in the role as psychotherapist? *Body, Movement and Dance in Psychotherapy*. DOI: doi:10.1080/17432979.2018.143079.

Brazelton, T. B., Koslowski, B., & Main, M. The origins of reciprocity: The early mother-infant interaction. In Lewis, M. & Rosenblum, L. A. (1974) *The effect of the infant on its caregiver*. Oxford: Wiley-Interscience.

Caldwell, C. (2017). Conscious movement sequencing: The core of the dance movement psychotherapy experience. In Payne, H. (Ed.). *Essentials of dance movement psychotherapy: International perspectives on theory, research and practice*. (pp. 53–66). London: Routledge.

Heller, M. C. (2012). *Body psychotherapy: History, concepts and methods*. New York: W.W. Norton.

Hesse, E. & Main, M. (1999). Second-Generation effects of unresolved trauma as observed in non-maltreating parents: Dissociated, frightened and threatening parental behaviour. *Psychoanalytic Inquiry*, 19, 481–540.

Janet, P. (1929). *L'Evolution psychologique de la personalité*. Paris: Chahine.

Laban, R. & Lawrence, F. C. (1974). *Effort*. London: MacDonald and Evans.

Lowen, A. (1973). *Depression and the body. The biological basis of faith and reality*. London: Penguin.

Lyons-Ruth, K. (1998). Implicit relational knowing: Its role in development and psychoanalytic treatment. *Infant Mental Health Journal*, 19, 282–289.

Main, M. & Solomon, J. (1986). Discovery of an insecure-disorganized/disoriented attachment pattern. In T. Berry, T. B. Brazelton, & Michael W. Yogman (Eds.). *Affective development in infancy* (pp. 95–124). Westport, CT: Ablex Publishing.

Marcher, L. & Fich, S. (2010). *Body encyclopedia: A guide to the psychological functions of the muscular system*. Berkeley, CA: North Atlantic Books.

Marks-Tarlow, T. (2013). *Clinical intuition in psychotherapy: The neurobiology of embodied response*. New York: W.W. Norton.

McGilchrist, I. (2009). *The master and his emissary: The divided brain and the making of the Western world*. New Haven, CT: Yale University Press.

Ogden, P., Minton, K., & Pain, C. (2006). *Trauma and the body: A sensorimotor approach to psychotherapy*. New York: W.W. Norton.

Porges, S. W. (2011). *The Polyvagal theory: Neurophysiological foundations of emotions, attachment, communication, and self-regulation*. New York: W.W. Norton.

Rosenberg, J. Lee., Rand, M. L., & Asay, D. (1985). *Body, self and soul sustaining integration*. Atlanta, Georgia: Humanics Limited.

Rothschild, B. (2000). *The body remembers: The psychophysiology of trauma and trauma treatment*. New York: W.W. Norton.

Rothschild, B. (2017). *The body remembers: Volume 2: Revolutionizing trauma treatment*. New York: W.W. Norton.

Schore, A. N. (1994). *Affect regulation and the origin of the self: The neurobiology of emotional development*. Mahwah, NJ: Erlbaum.

Schore, A. N. (2003). The seventh annual John Bowlby Memorial Lecture. Minds in the making: attachment, the self-organizing brain, and developmentally-oriented psychoanalytic psychotherapy. In J. Corrigall & H. Wilkinson (Eds.). *Revolutionary connection. Psychotherapy and neuroscience* (pp. 7–51). London: Karnac.

Schore, A. N. (2009). Right brain affect regulation: An essential mechanism of development, trauma, dissociation, and psychotherapy. In D. Fosha, D. J. Siegel, & M. F. Solomon (Eds.). *The healing power of emotion. Affective neuroscience, development, and clinical practice.* (pp. 112–144). New York: W.W. Norton.

Sletvold, J. (2014). *The embodied analyst: From Freud to Reich to relationality*. London: Routledge.

Southwell, C. (1988). The Gerda Boyesen Method: Biodynamic therapy. In J. Rowan & W. Dryden (Eds.). *Innovative therapy in Britain.* (pp. 178–201). Milton Keynes, UK: Open University Press.

Southwell, C. (2010). Levels of consciousness and contact in biodynamic psychotherapy. *The Psychotherapist*, Winter 2010, 10–11.

Trevarthen, C. (2009). The functions of emotion in infancy: The regulation and communication of rhythm, sympathy, and meaning in human development. In D. Fosha,

D. J. Siegel, & M. F. Solomon (Eds.). *The healing power of emotion: Affective neuroscience, development, and clinical practice.* (pp. 55–85). New York: W.W. Norton.

van der Kolk, B. (1994). The body keeps the score. *Harvard Review of Psychiatry, 1,* 253–265.

van der Kolk, B. (2014). *The body keeps the score: Mind, brain and body in the transformation of trauma.* London: Penguin.

Westland, G. (2015). *Verbal and non-verbal communication in psychotherapy.* New York: W.W. Norton.

Chapter 6

Psychodrama and healing the traumatic wound

Anna Chesner

The power of perspective

According to van der Kolk "[w]e are on the verge of becoming a trauma-conscious society." (van der Kolk, 2014, p. 347) The shift in consciousness to which he refers has been driven in part by new technology highlighting what goes on in the brain and how the brain and body are linked. Alongside this new data have come new perspectives on the therapeutic treatment of trauma and in particular the importance of an experiential approach that works not only top down from the mind to body but also bottom up from the body to the mind. Of key importance is the work of Daniel Siegel (e.g. Siegel, 2015), Peter Levine (e.g. Levine, 2010), and Pat Ogden (e.g. Ogden, Minton, & Pain, 2006), all of whom pay attention to the mind-body relationship and an experiential approach to working with trauma.

Of particular relevance are the mechanisms in the sympathetic nervous system when facing danger or perceived danger: the fight, flight, freeze response. The lower parts of the brain and brain stem bypass the higher functions of the prefrontal cortex and react to danger stimuli with an immediacy that higher brain functions cannot manage. In many ways this is useful for survival, but these same mechanisms mean that traumatic experiences may remain unprocessed for many years as clients react to stimuli in everyday life without understanding what is happening in their body/mind. Ways of being that were once survival strategies become embedded and automatic. Such patterns influence how we experience the world and our style of relating with others. In psychodramatic language our "role repertoire" becomes diminished, our spontaneity and creativity levels blocked, and the reciprocal role relationships we find ourselves in tend to reinforce negative and defensive beliefs we hold about our self, others, and the world. My use of the word belief here is not so much to do with consciously held and verbally articulated philosophical world views, but something more implicit, linked to procedural memory and somatic patterns of breath, posture, gesture, and facial expression.

Because the impact of trauma is profoundly connected to the interplay of body and mind, the therapies of choice are those which have their foundations in this very interplay. Psychodrama psychotherapy is one of these, based in the body, mind, senses, and imagination. Developed by J. L. and Zerka Moreno in the twentieth century its approach sits well with the current trauma consciousness to which van der Kolk refers.

In this chapter I link the three phases of trauma work outlined by Judith Herman (Herman, 1997) to the practice of psychodrama psychotherapy. I draw attention to a particular therapeutic feature of psychodrama psychotherapy; the experience of changing perspective, guided by the director. I reflect on how this supports the working through of trauma. I illustrate this through an example of a classical psychodrama, which is included here with the consent of the protagonist. Certain identifying features have been changed and omitted for purposes of confidentiality.

The three stages Herman (1997) outlines for all trauma work are Safety, Remembrance and Mourning, and Reconnection. I begin by asking what creates the foundation of safety and relationship in group psychodrama psychotherapy? This is an important question, as psychodrama is an impactful method, which must be used in an informed and mindful way. As with other experiential psychotherapies there has been a shift away from the approach of the seventies and eighties where there was an emphasis on emotional catharsis as the agent of change. Modern approaches to the method give as much attention to the therapeutic use of the imagination and the reflective function alongside the emotional aspects of the work (Napier & Chesner, 2014). Psychodrama is a holistic and integrative psychotherapy.

There follow some key principles to the establishment and maintenance of safety.

- **Attunement to individual and group.** An attuned relationship is paramount in all therapeutic endeavours, and especially where the impact of trauma makes participants vulnerable to dissociation or aggression if they feel overwhelmed by the work. In the group setting the therapist needs to be attuned both to the needs of the individual protagonist, whose work is the focus, and also to the group. He or she needs to develop a moment-to-moment awareness of the group, and may at times pause the action on the therapeutic stage in order to attend to what is happening in the group.
- **Group contract.** A clear group working contract gives reassurance to group members around their own agency. This is negotiated in the early stages of group formation. The group contract supports a working alliance and cohesion in the group, which is vital to all psychodrama, and especially so in the case of working with trauma material. Principles include the right to say no to a role anyone is asked to hold on stage as auxiliary. If a role is likely to be overwhelming, or if it is a role that is overdeveloped in the group member, exercising this right can be understood as an act of therapeutic self-care. Other helpful factors in the group contract are the commitment to regular and punctual attendance, and to stay in the room

during the session; in particular to make sure to return to the group the following session if the group member has done a piece of protagonist work – the group is invested in knowing the impact of the piece of work and how the protagonist is doing.

- **Pace.** It is essential to manage the pace of the group's work in the light of the levels of defence and anxiety in the group. This tends to mean going slowly at first, and the therapist/s not being in a hurry to move the work into challenging areas too quickly. The therapist needs to be alongside the group rather than ahead of them, laying the foundations of group cohesion and familiarity with the psychodramatic techniques before engaging with deeply explorative pieces of work. At times this may mean holding some individuals back from a tendency to race impulsively into their trauma work.

- **Session structure.** A predictable session structure contributes greatly to a sense of safety and trust. I think in terms of a five-phase structure: check-in, warm-up, action, sharing, and closure. The *check-in* is an opportunity for each person to arrive in the group and share verbally. I favour clear guidance as to what is to be shared, for example, something that is left over from last session, how you arrived today, and how your week has been; then that person invites someone else in the group to check in. This kind of check-in structure allows time for each person, but also encourages focus, so that people do not become too anxious that one person is dominating the process. The *warm-up* phase is an opportunity to engage the body and begin to move into playful action. Here too I favour a predictable structure such as standing up and creating a circle, making eye contact, saying the name of someone in the group, and throwing them a soft ball; or a sound and movement game. Typically, these warm-ups change the energy in the group, the body is activated, people start to breathe more fully, and there is eye contact and social engagement. Such a warm-up may be perceived as "silly" in the first instance but a degree of shared silliness can help ease habitual anxiety, and contribute to group bonding. The central phase of the group process is called the *action* phase, and this is where psychodramatic methods are used to explore current issues, past memories, future plans or strategies, and the development of more functional ways of being. This is often the most intense part of the process, and can focus at times on the group as a whole, or several individuals doing short explorations with the help of the group, or one individual working as a protagonist for a fuller exploration and working through of an issue, as we see in the example (see p. 74). The action is always followed by the final phase of the group, namely de-roling, role feedback, and *sharing*. This final phase is quite structured, and emphasises the here and now as a place to reflect back on the experience of the work and its impact on each individual. While the action phase inhabits the world of the psychodramatic stage, the sharing phase is rooted firmly in the present. We move away from the "as if"

(Kellerman, 2000, p. 111) of the stage where we have travelled in time to the past and future, and made visible the inner world of the protagonist. Through the sharing we return to a place of verbal reflection. Group members are encouraged as far as possible to name what they are in touch with in terms of their own memories, identifications and experiences as a result of witnessing the work on the stage, or holding a role for the protagonist. This is an important preparation for moving back out into everyday life and should be given plenty of time.

- **Working in bite-sized pieces.** Psychodrama can be an immensely powerful method. In order not to overwhelm clients who, by virtue of their trauma history, may be susceptible to overwhelm or not in touch with their own need for boundaries, it is advisable to introduce the method with shorter pieces of work. This allows several people to be the protagonist within one session, and plenty of time for de-roling and the sharing phase of the work. Each short exploration, through symbolisation, encounter or brief role reversal is immersive, but less so than a full classical psychodrama, which characteristically lasts approximately two hours. If participants know that the expectation for immersive engagement with their trauma, whether by being a protagonist or by witnessing the work of another group member, will be negotiated with a consideration of what is manageable, there is a good foundation for trust. The principle is one of dipping a toe in the water rather than being asked to dive straight in from the high board.

- **Specific focus for each piece of work.** A clear working contract for any particular piece of psychodrama work that is negotiated between the protagonist and the director is crucial. Such a contract makes explicit the intention of any piece of work. I tend to write this up on a flipchart so that it can be held in mind at any point. If the work becomes uncomfortable we can remind ourselves what our purpose is, and keep ourselves on track with that purpose. We do not find ourselves in an uncomfortable place for the gratification of the therapist, but for the purpose of addressing an agreed goal. A good contract is doable within the time frame of the session and appropriate to the level of familiarity with the method, the phase of the therapy, and the capacity of the group to support the work.

- **Prescriptive roles.** We have many roles or ways of being. Before approaching deep trauma work it is really helpful to resource the protagonist. Kate Hudgins in her Therapeutic Spiral Model (Kellerman, 2000; Hudgins, 2001, p. 237) outlines three kinds of prescriptive role that can be incorporated into a psychodrama at the beginning. The director asks the protagonist to identify a personal quality, interpersonal relationship, or transpersonal role that would support them to manage what is likely to be difficult work. Personal qualities might be courage, determination, capacity for love, commitment to change. Interpersonal relationships may include a good friend, a teacher, partner or role model from the public arena. Transpersonal roles might come from the realm of nature (the sun, mother earth, the cosmos) or from a faith meaningful to the protagonist (Jesus, Buddha, God). Before embarking on addressing the contracted theme, one of these roles is brought onto the stage. The protagonist reverses roles with them, accessing the particular quality of the role, and has a short conversation with them, negotiating how near they need them to be during the work, and any key words they need to hear from them. This simple prelude to the psychodrama often creates a visible and tangible change in the protagonist's demeanour as they approach the work. It is an impressive means of diminishing anxiety and helping the protagonist access their innate creativity and optimism. At times during the work where the protagonist is at the edge of their window of tolerance, in danger of shutting off or giving up on themselves (Siegel, 1999, cited in Ogden, et al., 2006) a brief role reversal with one of these prescriptive roles can support the protagonist to continue. Their perspective changes from overwhelmed victim to someone with access to an active resource. Since these roles are held by group members chosen by the protagonist for the task this technique also enables the group to give direct support to their fellow group member.

- **The double.** Trauma experiences are fundamentally ones of disconnection, from sensory experience, higher function thought, and interpersonal connection. The psychodramatic technique of the double can be useful to maintain connection with the here and now, to the senses, body, thought, and awareness of the other. The example that follows highlights the value of creating and maintaining social connectedness through this technique. Hudgins (ibid., p. 237) outlines further specialist uses of the double in trauma work, including the containing double, and body double.

Remembrance, working through, and the power of perspective

Having looked at some of the psychodrama-specific ways of fostering a climate of safety we now move on to the work of what Herman (1997) refers to as remembrance and mourning. Working through the impact of traumatic experiences is an act of remembering and meaning-making in the present. Trauma and dissociation involve not being present to the moment, because the moment of trauma was unbearable, and the hippocampus tends to go offline at such moments. The body and the senses, however, do hold important memories and as we step onto the psychodrama stage these fragmented experiences can begin to become integrated into consciousness, especially as we pay attention to moment-to moment changes in the protagonist's way of being.

A particular feature of psychodrama psychotherapy is the moving between perspectives, not just mentally but also in terms of our physical embodied experience. The basic building block of the method is *role reversal*. This is not just a mental or imaginative activity. Each role has its place on the stage, so each role reversal brings with it a literal change of perspective on the scene as the protagonist moves to a different position on the stage. A protagonist will be directed not only to reverse roles, but also at key moments to step outside of the scene into the reflective *mirror* position. This involves witnessing the scene that has been built up on the stage, perhaps from the perspective of a key object within the scene (a mirror, a tree, the light bulb) or from the audience space of the psychodrama, from the here and now of the therapy room. At other moments, particularly between one scene and another, or one memory and another, the protagonist and director pace around the perimeter of the stage area, in reflective dialogue. Pacing together in an attuned way, while reflecting out loud on what has been revealed so far and how it relates to the contract, offers a powerful grounding in the present as well as a pre-paration to re-enter the "as if" of the psychodramatic stage. I often ask the protagonist to make eye contact with the group during their work, so that the focus returns to the here and now of the session. Whether reversing roles, moving into the mirror position, or pacing in the here and now of the group session, the protagonist's perspective on the work keeps changing. The inter-play of these perspectives serves to loosen the rigidity that we can all experi-ence in terms of our sense of self, and our assumptive unconscious beliefs about self, other, and the world. Where there is a trauma response, our unconscious rigidity tends to be more pronounced. In psychodramatic terms our capacity for role flexibility is diminished and our spontaneity levels reduced as we try to keep ourselves "safe" in ways that perpetuate our fear, defensiveness, and isolation in relation to our world. Through these changes of perspective, protagonists can explore the boundaries of their window of tolerance, moving at times deeply into the experience as well as accessing their reflective function and their capacity to make sense of the experience in new and updated ways from an aesthetic distance.

Peter's psychodrama

Peter is chosen by the group to be protagonist. This piece of work is the cul-mination of four or five significant psychodramas over the course of a year or more all of which belong to the realm of relational trauma. His contract on this occasion is "I want to be able to trust that people like me for who I am and not for what I do." We can see from this contract that Peter has an awareness that there is something blocking his way of being with people he is close to. The contract itself points to the impact of early life experiences on Peter's ability to let the other in and to enjoy what is on offer in his life. While this piece of work is not about trauma as a single incident it is about the traumatic impact of growing up in an emotionally damaging environment.

Typically, we begin by setting up on the stage and enacting a recent example of the issue, a *presenting scene*. In this case Peter takes us to his home where his partner affectionately opens her arms to offer an embrace. As he moves towards her he notices an involuntary physical movement, whereby his arms cross over his own chest, forming a protective barrier between them. The body is doing something that makes no sense to his mind. Through role reversal he experiences both the role of his partner, affectionately offering a hug, as well as his own, apparently incongruous role response. In addition to the external reality of the scene, psychodrama allows us to bring onto the stage internal role responses, which are fleshed out in terms of their gesture, posture, and placement in relation to the protagonist, and these roles are then held by other group members. In this case we bring on to the stage an internal message that tells him "She must want something from you, be careful or you will be taken advantage of, exploited." As well as the internal roles we also mark on the stage the transference aspect of this recent scene. As he views the open arms of his partner, and hears the internal message of hypervigilant mistrust, he is aware of an association from the past, which we concretise on the stage. It is as if he is facing mother and father, whose messages are "Be how I need you to be, the way I know is good for you!" and "You will be consistently either rewarded or punished according to your compliance with my expectations and rules!" respectively. These messages from the past seem to be intruding at a physical level on his capacity to accept the love and closeness that is on offer in his current life. The scene is like a double exposure photograph – a recent moment, but with the intrusion of past relational elements that skew his experience of the present.

In order to make sense of what we witness on the stage I use role analysis to link what we are seeing on the stage to the contract. This formulation serves as the through line to give coherence to the different scenes brought on to the stage. There are five elements to role analysis: the *context* of the role, *behaviour*, *feelings*, implicit *belief*, and *consequences*. In this case we see that in a *context* of being offered affection by a significant other his *behaviour* is to externally comply partially, but internally to shut off and defend. He *feels* suspicious and bewildered. His implicit, embodied *belief* is that the other must want something from him, that his integrity could be compromised or overwhelmed, perhaps that there is no such thing as unconditional love. The *consequence* for him is that he remains defended and unable to give himself over to the love that is on offer.

In a brief second scene, whose purpose is to confirm, revise or fine tune this role analysis, he is invited to take us to a similar context, another situation where he is offered affection by someone he is close to. Here he is offered a hug by his adult son, as spontaneous thanks for a kindness Peter has done him. We see him receiving this hug with one arm only, his physical response betraying his ambivalence and unease. He is in a double bind, the best way he knows to show his love is through doing, but if he is affectionately thanked for that it means to him that he is only loved for what he can do.

In classical psychodrama we track the belief that has become incongruent in the present back to the situation or situations where it was the best or only response possible. This *locus* scene is often in childhood, a time when the protagonist was developing his internal working model (Bowlby, 1997). Sometimes this is a single event, at other times it is an exploration of a less tangible dynamic that is nonetheless formative. In Peter's case it is an early memory that is emblematic of the double bind described above. It is one of innumerable instances where he learns to view himself as needing to do or achieve in order to be loved, but also that any signs of love that are achieved in this way need to be defended against. Before we look at this scene, a few words about the process of his spontaneously accessing this memory and the part that the group plays in this.

Peter is a highly intelligent person, aware intellectually after several experiences of the method of how it works, but with a marked tendency to need to control the process, to think it through rather than let go into it. In other words, he struggles to give himself over to the flow and the spontaneity of the method much as he struggles to give himself over to a hug.

As psychodrama director I am aware of this, and experience myself as working hard to direct him in such a way that he can fully enter the experience. I am also aware of the group energy dropping. One person even appears to be nodding off. The most helpful principle in moments like this for me is "trust the group." So, at the end of the second scene, I pause the action, name what I am noticing and ask if there might be some group members who could *double* Peter, i.e. to come onto the stage, take on his physical position next to him, and to try and put into words in the first person as Peter what he is feeling, and what sense he is making of the scene we have witnessed. After each doubling statement I check with him if it is accurate and invite him to put it into his own words if it fits, and to dismiss it if not. It is an act of group mentalisation, an attempt at profound empathy on the part of the group members, who literally have to get up onto their feet and place themselves alongside him in a physical act of solidarity. They lend themselves to his ego as they offer to put their sense of his felt state into words. Moreno links the technique of doubling to the earliest mother infant relationship, where the mother attempts to feel with and articulate what is going on for baby before it has the capacity to use words. This involves the process Siegel refers to as alignment (cited in Ogden, Minton, & Pain, 2006 p.44). As director, I notice Peter sinking into his own experience, relaxing into the process of receiving offers of help and being connected with others. It is out of this process that a very early memory pops up for him.

By the time we move into the *locus scene*, group and protagonist are fully engaged.

The locus takes place when the protagonist is under three. He is an only child, his parents having tried for ten years for a baby, and he is the recipient of all their hopes and expectations. Relevant to their way of being is that they had both been acutely impacted by war, mother having been displaced; father persecuted, wounded, and imprisoned. There is undoubtedly a transgenerational and wider social context dimension to the situation we explore. Their capacity to offer an emotionally appropriate environment to raise a child is significantly diminished.

The scene depicts Peter's father trying to persuade him to recite a poem he had learned into a tape recorder, and Peter fundamentally not wanting to, not wanting to perform, not wanting to be shown off to others, not wanting to be told what he wants. Father is not malevolent in this, but he is characteristically unattuned and focused on task, achievement, and doing, rather than the value of being, and being together. His model of bringing up his son is based entirely and systematically on rewarding compliance and achievement and making sure Peter pays the price of any non-compliance. There is no concept or sense of meeting his son where he is. On this occasion he bribes him with the promise of a trip to the zoo if he performs for the tape recorder. Peter complies, but with a feeling of betraying himself and having been coerced. Once father has left the room he begins to delete the recording, but stops himself as he does not want to lose the promised outing. He wants father's love, wants the trip to the zoo, but is hurt that father has ignored his protests and is exerting power rather than attuning to his son's own truth. Mother's implicit message at this point is that he should submit to whatever is required of him and put on a good show. Previous psychodramas have shown mother's style of parenting to be impatient, intrusive, and focused on how things seem rather than authentic relational connection. Peter's role response to the lack of attunement available to him from either parent, and in the absence of other relatives or siblings who might relativise this deficit, is the development of a determined self-sufficiency, a kind of hardening of something inside his core as he sits alone and retreats into himself.

At this point in a psychodrama a group member is chosen by the protagonist to take on the role of the little child, so that the protagonist can view the scene with the director from the mirror position, i.e. through the eyes of the adult self and from outside the scene. The purpose of this shift of perspective is to facilitate the reflective function and to link it with the felt experience of the scene. By viewing the scene together with the director Peter is able to identify the deficit of attunement he is experiencing at this formative time in his life. He is moved by the angry, frightened loneliness of the little boy in front of him, preparing himself for a life of self-sufficiency and mistrust. He is invited to intervene in the scene, to do something different with or for his child self. His impulse is to go into the scene as himself, an adult man, one who is himself a father, and to spend time with himself as a little boy.

My sense is that this is a moment when words will not be enough, and where they might even get in the way of authentic emotional connection. So, I give the instruction to not use words, but to find a way to just "be with" the little boy in front of him. He steps back into the scene and what follows is a non-verbal negotiation between Peter as an adult and the group member holding the role of the frozen or closed off little Peter. He sensitively sits with his young self, tentatively and playfully offers delicate hand-to-hand contact, checking out all the time what the child's response is. Gradually he moves towards offering an embrace and ends up holding and rocking his little self. No word is spoken, but the scene is riveting. I instruct the two to reverse roles and the group member who has now physically experienced Peter's way of tentatively making contact takes on the role of adult Peter, while Peter returns to the role of his child self. This is the role that needs healing, that holds the original relational wound. In this role he gets the chance to receive what he has just given. What we witness as a group at this point is how frightened and frozen that little child is, and how patiently the reparative adult role needs to approach him. It takes considerably longer to play the scene this way round, as, true to the role, he is initially reluctant and afraid to let the other in. Finally, he is in the arms of his adult self and sobs as his inner armour releases and his basic human need for attuned connection is met. As director, I support this in a physical way by briefly placing my hands onto the two group members in the embrace, but mostly my role here is to hold the space, and to give permission for them to take the time that this process needs. Again, at this moment the group plays a part, through their supportive witnessing. The intervention is as moving as it is simple, evocative of the story of Warming the Stone Child, a traditional Inuit tale told by Clarissa Pinkola Estes (1990). The experience serves to contradict the rigidly held belief in his aloneness, and that there is no such thing as freely given and attuned affection.

All psychodramas conclude in the present, the only place where change can be lived. In Peter's case there is a brief return to the first scene, which is replayed. This time he finds himself able to respond spontaneously to the offer of an embrace from his partner. This "role training" scene is the first step towards testing the new internal role and integrating the work into his everyday life. Something has shifted.

Reconnection

In the final stage of a psychodrama session the enactment is followed by personal sharing by the group members. The process is one of reconnecting with the group in the here and now. The emotional resonance of the group is an important validation for the protagonist. In terms of Herman's three stages of trauma work it is part of the Reconnection phase of the work. Being a protagonist feels like a deep and intensely personal journey. Hearing the sharing of others in response to putting our own inner world on the stage mitigates against potential feelings of shame. It is also therapeutic for group members whether they have held a role on the psychodramatic stage or simply witnessed the work from the audience space to identify what personal memories and feelings have come up for them during the work. These resonances may form the seed for future pieces of protagonist work for them.

Reconnection is an ongoing process. For some weeks after Peter's work he reported a physical sensation of something in his core having shifted. He experienced a certain unfamiliarity to his sense of himself in the world, which was "not unpleasant" and which was hard to put into words. Comments he received from work colleagues, friends, and his partner validated that sense of something having changed in his way of being and relating.

As I read this chapter to him he is deeply moved, saying "I am re-experiencing my psychodrama, but from the perspective of the audience. These tears are sadness for that little boy, but also joy that something has shifted since the piece of work."

References

Bowlby, J. (1997). *Attachment Vol. 1 (Attachment and Loss)*. London: Random House.

Estes, C. P. (1997). *Warming the stone child: Myths and stories about abandonment and the unmothered child* (Audio CD). Sounds True.

Herman, J. (1997). *Trauma and recovery*. New York: Basic Books.

Hudgins, M. K. (2001). The therapeutic spiral model: Treating PTSD in action. In P. F. Kellerman & M. K. Hudgins (Eds.) *Psychodrama with trauma survivors*. London: Jessica Kingsley.

Kellerman, P. F. (2000). *Focus on psychodrama*. London: Jessica Kingsley.

Levine, P. (2010). *In an unspoken voice: How the body releases trauma and restores goodness*. Berkeley, CA: North Atlantic Books.

Napier, A. & Chesner, A. (2014) Psychodrama and mentalization, loosening the illusion of a fixed reality. In P. Holmes, M. Farrall, K. Kirk (Eds.) *Empowering therapeutic practice*. London: Jessica Kingsley.

Ogden, P., Minton, K. & Pain, C. (2006). *Trauma and the body*. New York: W.W. Norton.

Siegel, D. (2015). *The developing mind: How relationships and the brain interact to shape who we are*. New York: Guilford Press.

van der Kolk, B. (2014). *The body keeps the score*. London: Penguin Random House.

Chapter 7

Building resilience

Developing embodied and relational resources in a Gestalt movement therapy group

Yeva Feldman

This chapter interweaves theory, research, and clinical applications of a Gestalt movement therapy (GMT) group for women diagnosed with borderline personality disorder (BPD) who have experienced profound trauma. The GMT group, an experiential movement group, combining Gestalt therapy (GT) and dance movement psychotherapy (DMP), emphasised bodily and social re-connection (Feldman 2016, 2017). It took place on a specialist BPD inpatient unit utilising Linehan's (1993) dialectical behaviour therapy (DBT) framework, a cognitive-behavioural approach specifically designed for treating BPD. There are a growing number of approaches highlighting the centrality of the body in treating trauma (e.g. Buckley, Punkanen, & Ogden, 2018; Federman & Sterenfeld, 2017; Kepner, 1995; Levine, 2005; Ogden, Minton, & Pain, 2006; Rothschild, 2002; van der Kolk, 2014), as well as in working with BPD (e.g. Delisle, 1999; Lavendar & Sobelman, 1995; Lopez, 2011; Warnecke, 2009). Trauma has a long-lasting impact on adult experience (Herman, 1992; Harms, 2015) and takes away the sense of power (agency), control and the capacity to respond physically in the moment (Herman, 1992; Kepner, 1995; Levine, 2005; Ogden et al., 2006; van der Kolk, 2014). Movement is inherently dynamic and promotes self-agency and control. Working relationally with movement can help develop and fortify somatic resilience, which is essential in recovery from trauma (Buckley et al., 2018; Federman & Sterenfeld, 2017; Kepner, 1995; Joyce & Sills, 2014; Ogden et al., 2006; Taylor, 2014; van der Kolk, 2014). This chapter will address the specific needs and treatment considerations when working with trauma in relation to this client group, illustrating the role and importance of movement in building resilience through strengthening relational and embodied resources.

BPD and trauma: the connection

It is often difficult to distinguish between post-traumatic stress disorder (PTSD) and BPD especially when there is a history of early trauma (Woodward, Gordon, Taft, & Meis, 2009). Trauma is highly prevalent in those diagnosed with BPD and this client group reported the highest rate of traumatic events compared to those with other mental health disorders (Yen, Shea, Battle, Johnson, Zlotnick, Dolan-Sewell, et al., 2002). Some believe that the diagnosis of BPD is due to the individual's response to underlying trauma (Cavazzi & Becerra, 2014; van der Kolk, 2014); 90 per cent of individuals with BPD experienced early trauma in the form of parental maltreatment (physical abuse, neglect) and 75 per cent have a history of childhood sexual abuse (Kaehler & Freyd, 2012). In addition, 75 per cent of patients diagnosed with BPD are women (Gunderson & Links, 2008).

The high incidence of "attachment trauma," trauma that occurs within the context of the primary attachment relationship (Harms, 2015, p. 54) in individuals with BPD, suggests that this is a distinguishing precursor to the disorder (Yen, et al., 2014). There are adverse and long-term effects of such trauma on the individual's capacity to develop and maintain relationships and regulate internal states (Harms, 2015; van der Kolk, 2014). Early attachment trauma is linked with depression, hopelessness, suicide, a sense of emptiness, identity disturbance, confusion, dissociation, and emotional dysregulation. This may explain why these symptoms are greater in individuals with BPD than in any other mental health disorders (Marco, Perez, Garcia-Alandete, & Moliner, 2015).

Treatment implications

Although there is a similar presentation found between BPD and PTSD, namely a high incidence of self-harm and suicidality (Woodward, et al., 2009), the focus of the treatment is significantly different. Both attachment and trauma need to be addressed. In BPD, treatment of emotional dysregulation, dissociation, and interpersonal problems may need to be addressed first due to the severity of functional impairment and suffering (Kaehler & Freyd, 2012). As the incidence of completed suicide is 50 per cent greater among individuals with BPD (Oldham, 2006), suicidal and intentional self-injurious behaviours are a high priority for inpatient treatment (Bohus, Haaf, Simms, Limberger, Schmahl, Unckel, et al., 2004).

It is widely accepted that this is a complex and challenging group of clients to treat. Clinically, the diagnosis of BPD is contentious and prone to misconceptions and stigma that may negatively affect clients' treatment (Woodward, et al., 2009). Clients prefer the updated name of "emotionally unstable personality disorder" (EUPD) for this reason (Mind, 2018). The diagnosis of BPD is in fact a description of symptoms and the starting point, rather than the complete story (Delisle, 1999).

Biosocial model of BPD

BPD reflects a pattern of behavioural, emotional, and cognitive instability, and dysregulation, which impacts all aspects of the individual's life (APA, 2013; Linehan, 1993; Delisle, 1999). Linehan's (1993) biosocial model identifies emotional dysregulation as the core difficulty for BPD. It suggests that there is a biological predisposition of an oversensitive and over-reactive emotional response system. The combination of the inability to modulate and self-soothe physiological arousal with an invalidating environment produces the symptoms associated with BPD (Linehan, 1993). However, psychophysiological studies found hypoarousal and not hyperarousal when measuring physiological parameters associated with the fight and flight response in BPD (Cavazzi & Becerra, 2014). Research investigating the influence of past trauma appears to indicate that it is the trauma history rather than the BPD diagnosis, that may explain the theorised hyperreactivity, and potential behavioural impulsivity in BPD (Cavazzi & Becerra, 2014). Consequently, the current biosocial theory (Linehan, 1993) may not adequately describe everyone diagnosed with BPD, rather only a subtype strongly associated with dissociation and a history of trauma (Cavazzi & Becerra, 2014).

Resilience

Resilience is the capacity and resourcefulness to "bounce back" from adversity (Harms, 2015, p. 10). It relates to the capacity of the individual to use resources that sustain well-being (Harms, 2015). Resilience is both innate and learnt (Buckley, et al., 2018). Individuals with BPD combined with histories of trauma demonstrate less resilience than other individuals with different mental health disorders (Marco, et al., 2015). Bearing pain and distress skilfully is an essential goal for mental health (Linehan, 1993a) and crucial for building resilience (Lopez, 2011). The acquisition of skills and positive resources will strengthen resilience and the ability to respond to future stressors and crises adaptively, flexibly, and effectively (Joyce & Sills, 2014; Graham, 2013; Linehan, 1993).

Movement inherently promotes an experience of freedom and flexibility. While moving, clients can choose creative options and explore novel alternatives. Moving freely and authentically reinforces body ownership and agency. This in turn supports the experience of safety and trust in their bodies (Federman & Sterenfeld, 2017). Positive affect and satisfaction are natural derivatives of moving authentically with others (Feldman, 2017). Movement within the therapeutic relationship fosters development of new skills and resources, which boost resilience.

The setting

The GMT group took place on a specialist inpatient psychiatric unit for women diagnosed with BPD: a majority of the clients had histories of extreme and complex trauma, severe self-harm and numerous suicide attempts. Previous multiple and prolonged hospitalisations were common (e.g. up to ten years). Clients viewed this unit as their last chance for recovery as all other treatments had failed.

This two-year programme included a DBT "Psychosocial Skills Training" (Linehan, 1993a, p. 1) in the first year and a focus on trauma recovery in the second year. The programme was individualised as some clients needed longer in the first stage of the treatment. A multidisciplinary team consisting of DBT and trauma specialists provided necessary holding and treatment for this client group. This team understood that a positive, interpersonal, and collaborative relationship was crucial for therapeutic progress and reducing suicide (Linehan, 1993a).

An embodied relational approach

Dance movement psychotherapy is an embodied approach to psychotherapy, using movement and dance to promote well-being through the integration of physical, social, emotional, and cognitive functioning (Goodill, 2005). Although it is a psychotherapy approach in its own right, it is not uncommon to find theoretical eclecticism and integration in the field of DMP (Levy, 1988), for example with Gestalt therapy (GT), as illustrated here. GT is a humanistic, present-oriented approach aiming to activate awareness within a dialogic relationship (Perls, 1973; Hycner, 1995). Embodiment is the experience of having and being your body where there is no distinction between body and self-experience (Kepner, 2003). My approach centres around creating a potential space for embodiment to emerge within a dialogic relationship. An embodied dialogical relationship validates the uniqueness of each person and establishes mutuality and dialogue through words and movement (Chaiklin & Schmais, 1993; Hycner, 1995). Treatment needs to reactivate the capacity to safely mirror, and be mirrored by, others and to be truly heard and seen by another (Kepner, 1995). The integration of movement within a dialogical relationship has the potential to repair "attachment trauma" (Harms, 2015, p. 54) through non-verbal attunement, mirroring, and validation.

Group modality

A group approach with this client group supports the development of interpersonal skills and social support. An important aspect of mental health is being able to feel safe with other people (van der Kolk, 2014). The GMT group provided an opportunity for clients to experience safety and develop trust with others non-verbally, through movement. Developing their "relational intelligence" (Graham, 2013, p. xxix) and cultivating a sense of commonality and belonging (Yalom, 1985) in the group were all steps towards building a supportive community necessary for recovery (Langmuir, Kirsh, & Classen, 2011; Joyce & Sills, 2014; van der Kolk, 2014). In addition, a group approach minimised the intense fluctuating transference of idealisation/degradation, which is commonly projected on individual therapists by this client group (Linehan, 1993a).

Developing relational resources

The backbone of all treatment and recovery for this client group is relational and social reconnection (Herman, 1992; Kepner, 1995; van der Kolk, 2014). Social support is not just important, it is a "biological necessity" (van der Kolk, 2014, p. 167). In the GMT group, relational support was strengthened through the process of embodiment, mirroring, and symbolic movements. When a group member initiated an authentic "action" of self-expression, the movement was physically mirrored by the rest of the group. The meaning of the individual's movement was understood implicitly and explicitly through embodiment and words. "Body actions" (Chace, 1993, p. 207) can symbolically express a feeling or a need; for example, a reaching out movement can symbolise a need for connection, or a stamping movement can symbolise anger. Explorations that use the "experience of movement, on both symbolic and expressive levels, can transform individuals and guide their journeys to recovery" (Berger, 1995, pp. ix–x). Mirroring and responding to each other's movements created a sense of affirmation and being known and felt by another (Kepner, 1995). In the GMT group, relational support was experienced and explored implicitly and explicitly through movement and words. This strengthened clients' abilities to recognise, accept, and give relational support, which inevitably fortified resilience.

Developing embodied resources

Resilience cannot simply be processed cognitively and emotionally. There is a need for an embodied experience of resilience, which "leads clients to greater integration and sense of unitary wholeness as an embodied being in the world" (Buckley, et al., 2018, p. 232). Developing embodied resources implies having access to your body experience and being able to acknowledge this as "self-experience" (Kepner, 2003, p. 12), intrinsic to who you are. It means developing body ownership and a sense of body/self-agency, which is often lost through trauma (Herman, 1992; Kepner, 1995). Specifically, for this client group, it involves experiencing one's body as a safe resource in its own right (Federman & Sterenfeld, 2017; Taylor, 2014); it means acknowledging existing survival resources, promoting self-regulation and agency by expanding underdeveloped bodily resources, and experiencing pleasure (Buckley et al., 2018; Kepner, 1995; Ogden et al., 2006; van der Kolk, 2014). The GMT group provided clients with a creative, playful and non-threatening space to consolidate an embodied experience of safety, self-regulation, and self-agency.

Early creative adaptations to endangerment are structured in our body tissue and neural pathways, profoundly shaping our bodily and self-experience (Kepner, 2003; van der Kolk, 2014); These adjustments should be validated for their role in survival of trauma and can then be strengthened and developed (Buckley et al., 2018). It is common for clients to feel betrayed by their bodies, and to distrust and attack their bodies (alcohol, drugs, self-harm) in an attempt to manage over-whelming distress and intrusive memories (Herman, 1992; Lavender & Sobelman,

1995; Taylor, 2014 van der Kolk, 2014). Fluctuating between experience of high arousal, dissociation, and numbness destabilises their sense of self and somatic ground (Kepner, 1995; Pierce, 2014). Consequently, specific attention needs to be paid to improving embodied resources, and the capacity to integrate and organise body experience (Buckley et al., 2018; Ogden, et al., 2006).

Physical functions, such as breathing, grounding, body boundaries, posture, and movement emerge from physical experience, yet support self-regulation and psychological health (Buckley et al., 2018; Kepner, 1995; Ogden et al., 2006). Just as our bodies can reveal our histories (Federman & Sterenfeld, 2017), change at a body level is associated with change in overall functioning (Levy, 1998). The experience of grounding and self-soothing are essential to coping with intense emotions and distress (Kepner, 1995). By physically experiencing and practising grounding and self-soothing, clients are better able to tolerate bodily sensations and use their bodies as a source of information, strength, and support (Langmuir et al., 2012; Graham, 2013; Joyce & Sills, 2014). In the GMT group, individual self-soothing movements were identified and explored, widening the group's repertoire of self-regulating methods.

Severely disorganised or dissociated individuals, however, may be unable to pay attention to body sensation or breathing without becoming further distressed and confused. Body interventions that directly address trauma may be experienced as deregulating and threatening. Attending to sensation, bodily responses and breathwork needs to proceed slowly and gently, at the client's pace and readiness to engage (Lopez, 2011; Ogden & Minton, 2000). In order to move, clients need to feel safe (Lavendar & Sobelman, 1995). The therapist needs to be able to judge the readiness of the group, and introduce and pace embodied interventions accordingly, while remaining relationally available (Kepner, 1995; Joyce & Sills, 2014). Building a supportive somatic ground and a sense of physical safety are vital first steps for recovery.

Group rhythmic movement

Immobilisation has been thought of as the root of most traumas (van der Kolk, 2014; Levine, 2005). In the GMT group, moving together to a steady rhythm enabled clients to mobilise and reconnect. "Rhythmically attuned movements can create a small safe place where social engagement systems could begin to re-emerge" (van der Kolk, 2014, p. 85). "Symbolic rhythmic action" (Chace, 1993, p. 263), movements that express a feeling or need embedded in a rhythmic beat, contain, clarify, and communicate group emotional expression. This is a naturally satisfying experience bringing together breath and action (Schmais, 1985). It supports development of empathy (Behrends, Muller, & Dziobek, 2012) as a means to reactivate the individual's capacity to safely mirror and be mirrored by others (Kepner, 1995). In the GMT group, clients expressed difficult emotions, and developed a sense of community and belonging through rhythmic movement.

The embodied therapist

The therapist's own experience of embodiment is intrinsic to, and holds an important role in, the healing relationship (Chaiklin & Wengrower, 2009; Kepner, 2003). The therapist listens, and registers what the client is saying and doing with her own body, which fosters a deeper understanding, containment, and communication with clients (Colace, 2017 Kepner, 2003). Embodied therapists replicate the client's internal and physical experience in their own body serving as a "psychobiological regulator" (Shore, 2003, p. 185), attuning to nonverbal cues, recognising and modulating somatic experience, and modelling self-regulation (Ogden et al., 2006; Schore, 2003). The therapist's capacity to self-regulate depends on how "anchored" she is within her own body (Carroll, 2009, p. 102). When the therapist models self-regulatory actions, group members experience the same actions even when not moving through the function of "embodied simulation" (Gallese, 2009, p. 527). Through the activation of mirror neurons, internal body states associated with self-regulation are evoked in the observer, as if she were performing a similar action and experiencing similar sensations (Gallese, 2009). Authentic and spontaneous movement is a mutually regulatory process allowing implicit and explicit elements of expression to emerge, whereby both client and therapist are collaboratively co-regulating and being impacted on a somatic level.

A composite group vignette

This vignette demonstrates the development of the group over the duration of a year. It does not highlight any specific client material but rather focuses on the whole group experience and process.

Individuals from the unit came in and sat on the floor with their backs against the wall in an open circle. I asked them to notice how the wall/floor supported them and modelled pushing gently into the wall/floor while exhaling to increase this awareness. They watched me and some tried it out for themselves, shifting their posture to a more upright position. Continuing on with a verbal check-in, each person said they didn't want to move. After validating this decision, they chatted about current affairs. When we had "warmed up" socially, I took out a few balls to gauge their response. A few leaned forward appearing interested. Initially they rolled the balls to each other, which developed into gentle ball throwing. The ball game became more playful and creative; they were more willing to experiment with different ways of passing the ball to each other, which provided energy and support for further interactions and exploration. Noticing the group's readiness, I suggested warming up physically, inviting each person to suggest a movement that was right for them today. Clients initiated movements from their periphery (hands and feet). I highlighted the variations of these movements by others in the group. I introduced the element of breath and supported the development of each movement as translated through my own body. Movements that had a self-soothing capacity (rocking, swaying, stretching, self-holding, curling up small, etc.) were expanded and repeated. After a few months, individuals felt safer in taking more "risks" when moving in space and made more contact with each other. Gradually they initiated more dynamic and expressive movements, utilised space and props, explored polarities, and worked more relationally. This enabled emotionally embedded movements to emerge. Using rhythmic movement action, repetition, and voice, emotions were acknowledged and expressed in a contained and safe way (Chace, 1993). Rhythm and voice became a central focus for the group. Leaning against a large physio ball, the group created an orchestra of voices, using their own bodies and voices to make rhythms. The group would wind down by listening and moving to soothing music and physically recapping any movements that were experienced as supportive. Most sessions ended with a relaxation, accompanied by soothing music, imagery, and breath. After the relaxation, we transitioned to a verbal check out, reorienting to the present time and space and reconnecting verbally as a group.

Reflective notes

In the GMT group, I took every opportunity to highlight environmental support whenever and however it emerged. The walls became part of the holding environment (Winnicott, 1971) that provided the group with a sense of safety and containment. By modelling the pushing against the wall with exhalation, the clients who were not actively participating could still experience a sense of grounding through the process of "embodied simulation" (Gallese, 2009, p. 527). Pacing, grading, and choices were essential ingredients in the GMT group, which allowed clients to become authors of their own recovery, and their power and control to be restored (Herman, 1992). Creative and playful exploration (ball game) implied the development of trust in the group (Winnicott, 1971). Paying attention to micro-movements and non-verbal cues was vitally important in the early phase of a session and group process, as these were often clues to their natural resources and unfinished expression. Individual movements, no matter how small, were mirrored by the group, demonstrating acceptance and validation of each member.

Clients were able to regulate the intensity of their bodily experience by chatting as they moved and by initiating movements from the periphery (hands, feet, head), which meant their core was not activated and remained protected (Kepner, 1995). Using my own embodied experience of their movements helped to identify and translate subtle non-verbal expressions of emotions into more satisfying expression supported by rhythmic movements (Chace, 1993). Connecting with others through rhythm, voice, and play enabled clients to experience relational support. Ending with gentle movements to soothing music and guided relaxation, allowed them to identify the sensations associated with self-care and feeling at ease (van der Kolk, 2014).

They experienced flexibility, crucial for recovery (van der Kolk, 2014), by expanding their movement range and exploring creative options; they made choices about how, when, and where they moved or remained still; they become active agents in control of their bodies; they moved spontaneously, integrating breath with movement to orient themselves to the present moment. Difficult feelings were safely expressed and contained through symbolic rhythmic movements (Chace, 1993). In these ways, the GMT group provided clients with moments in which they could reclaim and build positive resources in their bodies, strengthening their capacity for resilience.

Conclusion

An approach that is embodied, present-oriented, experiential, and relational is particularly well-suited to working with individuals with BPD who have histories of profound trauma. Working in a group modality, using non-verbal means of connection and expression, fosters the experience of belonging to a social community, necessary for recovery (Harms, 2015; van der Kolk, 2014). The GMT group combined movement, social engagement, and embodied methods of self-soothing to develop resources and support. Novel experiences are necessary for the establishment of new neurological pathways in order to build insight and resilience (Graham, 2013; Lavender & Sobelman, 1995). I have found that clients were more likely to engage and tolerate new body sensations while moving with others. Safety, empowerment, control, and re-connection were addressed through the moving relationship. This embodied experience in the GMT group enabled clients to move forwards, to regain essential bodily and relational resources and to become more resilient.

References

American Psychiatric Association. (2013). *Diagnostic and statistical manual of mental disorders* (5th edn.). Washington, DC: APA.

Behrends, A., Muller, S., & Dziobek, I. (2012). Moving in and out of synchrony: A concept for a new intervention fostering empathy through interactional movement and dance. *The Arts in Psychotherapy*, 39(2), 107–116. doi:10.1016/j.aip.2012.02.003.

Berger, M. (1995). Foreword. In F. J. Levy (Ed.), *Dance movement therapy: A healing art*. Reston, VA: American Alliance for Health, Physical Education, Recreation and Dance.

Bohus, M., Haaf, B., Simms, T., Limberger, M. F., Schmahl, C., Unckel, C., *et al.*, (2004). Effectiveness of inpatient dialectical behavioral therapy for borderline personality disorder: A controlled trial. *Behaviour, Research and Therapy*, 42(5), 487–499. doi:10.1016/S0005-7967(03)00174–00178.

Buckley, T., Punkanen, M., & Ogden, P. (2018). The role of the body in fostering resilience: A sensorimotor psychotherapy perspective. *Body, Movement and Dance in Psychotherapy: An International Journal for Theory, Research and Practice*, 13(4), 225–233. doi:10.1080/17432979.2018.1467344.

Carroll, R. (2009). Self-regulation – an evolving concept at the heart of body psychotherapy. In L. Hartley (Ed.), *Contemporary body psychotherapy: The Chiron approach* (pp. 89–105). New York: Routledge.

Cavazzi, T. & Becerra, R. (2014). Psychophysiological research of borderline personality disorder: Review and implications for biosocial theory. *Europe's Journal of Psychology*, 10(1), 185–203. https://ro.ecu.edu.au/ecuworkspost2013/215.

Chace, M. (1993). Techniques for the use of dance as a group therapy. In S. L. Sandel, S. Chaiklin & A. Lohn (Eds.), *Foundations of dance/ movement therapy: The life and work of Marian Chace* (pp. 204–209). Maryland: The Marian Chace Memorial Fund of the American Dance Therapy Association.

Chaiklin, S. & Schmais, C. (1993). The Chace approach to dance therapy. In S. L. Sandel, S. Chaiklin, & H. Wengrower, *The art and science of dance/movement therapy*. New York: Routledge.

Colace, E. (2017). Dance movement therapy and developmental trauma: Dissociation and enactment in a clinical case study. *Body, Movement and Dance in Psychotherapy. An International Journal for Theory, Research and Practice*, 12(1), 36–49. https://doi.org/10.1080/17432979.2016.1247115.

Delisle, G. (1999). *Personality disorders*. Montreal, Canada: CIG Press.

Federman, D. G. & Sterenfeld, G. Z. (2017). Overcoming trauma: When verbal language is not enough. In H. Payne (Ed.), *Essentials of dance movement psychotherapy: International perspectives on theory, research and practice* (pp. 171–186). New York: Routledge.

Feldman, Y. (2016). *How body psychotherapy influenced me to become a dance movement psychotherapist. Body, Movement and Dance in Psychotherapy: An International Journal for Theory, Research and Practice*, 11(2–3), 103–113. doi:10.1080/17432979.2015.1095802.

Feldman, Y. (2017). Gestalt and dance movement psychotherapy in adults with eating disorders: Moving towards integration through practice and research. In H. Payne (Ed.), *Essentials of dance movement psychotherapy: International perspectives on theory, research and practice* (pp. 83–98). New York: Routledge.

Gallese, V. (2009). Mirror neurons, embodied simulation and the neural basis of social identification. *Psychoanalytic Dialogues: The International Journal of Relational Perspectives*, 19(5), 519–536. doi:10.1080/10481880903231910.

Goodill, S. W. (2005). *An introduction to medical dance/movement therapy: Health care in motion*. Philadelphia, PA: Jessica Kingsley.

Graham, L. (2013). *Bouncing back: Rewiring your brain for maximum resilience and well-being*. Novato, CA: New World Library.

Gunderson, J. G. & Links, P. S. (2008). The borderline diagnosis. In J. G. Gunderson & P. S. Links (Eds.), *Borderline personality disorder. A clinical guide* (pp. 1–28). Washington, US: American Psychiatric Publishing.

Harms, L. (2015). *Understanding trauma and resilience*. London: Palgrave.

Herman, J. L. (1992). *Trauma and recovery: The aftermath of violence – from domestic abuse to political terror*. New York: Basic Books.

Hycner, R. (1995). The dialogic ground. In R. Hycner & L. Jacobs (Eds.), *The healing relationship in Gestalt therapy* (pp. 3–29). New York: The Gestalt Journal Press.

Joyce, P. & Sills, C. (2014). *Skills in Gestalt counselling & psychotherapy* (3rd edn.). London: Sage.

Kachler, L. A. & Freyd, J. J. (2012). Betrayal trauma and borderline personality characteristics: Gender differences. *Psychological Trauma: Theory, Research, Practice and Policy*, 4(4), 379–385. doi:10.1037/a0024928.

Kepner, J. I. (1995). *Healing tasks: Psychotherapy with adult survivors of childhood abuse*. San Francisco, US: Jossey-Bass.

Kepner, J. I. (2003). The embodied field. *The British Gestalt Journal*, 12(1), 6–14.

Langmuir, J. I., Kirsh, S. G., & Classen, C. C. (2012). A pilot study of body-oriented group psychotherapy: Adapting sensorimotor psychotherapy for the group treatment of trauma. *Psychobiological Trauma: Theory, Research, Practice, and Policy*, 4(2), 214–220. doi:10.1037/a0025588.

Lavendar, J. & Sobelman, W. (1995). "I can't have me if I don't have you": Working with borderline personality. In F. Levy (Ed.) *Dance and other expressive art therapies: When words are not enough* (pp. 69–83). New York: Routledge.

Levine, P. A. (2005). *Healing trauma: A pioneering program for restoring the wisdom of your body*. Boulder, CO: Sounds True.

Levy, F. J. (1988). *Dance movement therapy: A healing art*. Reston, VA: American Alliance for Health, Physical Education, Recreation and Dance.

Linehan, M. M. (1993). *Cognitive-behavioral treatment of borderline personality disorder*. New York: The Guilford Press.

Linehan, M. M. (1993a) *Skills training manual for treating borderline personality disorder*. New York: The Guilford Press.

Lopez, G. (2011). Why verbal psychotherapy is not enough to treat post-traumatic stress disorder: A biosystemic approach to stress debriefing. *Body, Movement and Dance in Psychotherapy. An International Journal for Theory, Research and Practice*, 6(2), 129–143. doi:10.1080/17432979.2011.583060.

Marco, J. H., Perez, S., Garcia-Alandete, J., & Moliner, R. (2017). Meaning in life in people with borderline personality disorder. *Clinical Psychology and Psychotherapy*, 24(1), 162–170. doi:10.1002/cpp.1991.

Mind (2018). Borderline personality disorder. Retrieved from www.mind.org.uk/information-support/types-of-mental-health-problems/borderline-personality-disorder-bpd.

Ogden, P. & Minton, K. (2000). Sensorimotor psychotherapy: One method for processing traumatic memory. *Traumatology*, 3(3), 149–173. doi:10.1177/153476560000600302.

Ogden, P., Minton, K., & Pain, C. (2006). *Trauma and the body: A sensorimotor approach to psychotherapy*. London: W.W. Norton.

Oldham, J. M. (2006). Borderline personality disorder and suicidality. *American Journal of Psychiatry*, 163(1), 20–26. doi:10.1176/appi.ajp.163.1.20.

Perls, F. S. (1973). *The Gestalt approach and eye witness to therapy*. New York: Bantam.

Pierce, L. (2014). The integrative power of dance/movement therapy: Implications for treatment of dissociation and developmental trauma. *The Arts in Psychotherapy*, 41, 7–15.

Rothschild, B. (2002). Body psychotherapy without touch: Application for trauma therapy. In T. Staunton (Ed.), *Body psychotherapy* (pp. 101–115). New York: Routledge.

Schmais, C. (1985). *The healing processes in group dance therapy. American Journal of Dance Therapy*, 8(1), 17–36. doi:10.1007/BF02251439.

Schore, A. N. (2003). *Affect dysregulation and disorders of the self*. New York: W.W. Norton.

Taylor, M. (2014). *Trauma therapy and clinical practice: Neuroscience, Gestalt and the body*. Maidenhead, UK: Open University Press.

van Der Kolk, B. (2014). *The body keeps the score: Mind, brain and body in the transformation of trauma*. London: Penguin Random House.

Warnecke, T. (2009). The borderline relationship. In L. Hartley (Ed.), *Contemporary body psychotherapy: The Chiron approach* (pp. 194–211). New York: Routledge.

Winnicott, D. W. (1971). *Playing and reality*. London: Routledge.

Woodward, H. E., Gordon, R. A., Taft, C. T., & Meis, L.A. (2009). Clinician bias in the diagnosis of posttraumatic stress disorder and borderline personality disorder. *Psychological Trauma: Theory, Research, Practice and Policy*, 1(4), 282–290. doi:10.1037/a0017944.

Yalom, I. D. (1985). *The theory and practice of group psychotherapy* (3rd ed.). New York: Basic Books.

Yen, S., Shea, M. T., Battle, C. L., Johnson, D. M., Zlotnick, C., Dolan-Sewell, R., *et al.*, (2002). Traumatic exposure and posttraumatic stress disorder in borderline, schizotypal, avoidant and obsessive-compulsive personality: Findings from the collaborative longitudinal personal disorders study. *The Journal of Nervous and Mental Disease*, 190(8), 510–518. doi:10.1097/01.NMD.0000026620.66764.78.

Chapter 8

Dance movement psychotherapy

The body tells the unspeakable

Marianne Eberhard-Kaechele

"The trauma came through my body and it must leave the same way." In over thirty years of clinical experience, I have repeatedly heard this message from patients who suffer from complex trauma, which Herman (1992) defines as long-term, repeated, interpersonal abuse, often beginning early in life. Of course, it is not that simple. Neither damaging nor healing in interpersonal trauma occur only through the body, but also through the mind and relationship patterns. However, the body is a central medium of expression of the mind and relationships, yet often missing as a factor in standard forms of psychotherapy for trauma. This chapter presents a selection of contributions that dance movement psychotherapy (DMP) can make to trauma treatment, considering theory and research findings, and illustrated by clinical vignettes.

Why words are not enough

This chapter explores four reasons why words are not enough for treating complex trauma. The first reason is that the predisposition for post-traumatic stress disorders often begins at a preverbal level, through early *dysregulated attachment experiences,* including abuse and neglect (Schore, 2014). The second reason is that *the body is the scene of the crime* of trauma and may retain remnants that remind the survivor of their torment, causing obsession with, denial or persecution of the body (Young, 1992). From this perspective, words are indeed not enough to enable healing. The third reason is that many trauma survivors are unable, rather than unwilling, to speak about and overcome their experiences, due to *peritraumatic dissociation.* Dissociation is an initially involuntary survival mechanism, which temporarily separates mind and body, and reduces brain functions to sensorimotor survival patterns of the amygdala, while the speech centres of the prefrontal cortex shut down (van der Kolk, 2015). The fourth reason is that *implicit negative representations of self and others,* resulting from enacted abuse or neglect, distort survivors' perception (Briere, 2002). This undermines the assimilation of positive new experiences expressed verbally and challenges us to find forms of conveying self-worth or safety beyond words.

Dance movement psychotherapy

One way of fostering healing beyond words is DMP. DMP assumes the interrelation of somatic, emotional, cognitive, and social processes, and can be defined as the psychotherapeutic use of dance and movement in an interactional process aimed at the treatment of illness and the development or maintenance of physical and psychological health and quality of life (Levy, 2005). Bernstein (1995, p. 42) says of DMP with traumatised patients: "In dance therapy the body becomes at once the vehicle for change and the focus of change, so that the client can begin to reclaim her body as an ally in her struggle toward health."

DMP uses specific methods, which originated in dance art and are particularly appropriate for the treatment of traumatised individuals. In this chapter the following methods will be highlighted:

- the therapeutic movement relationship
- movement analysis
- movement metaphor
- the choreographic process

Before specific DMP methods are described, important trans-methodological ground rules (Rothschild, 2002) are mentioned here: the therapeutic situation, including the therapeutic relationship, should be transparent, safe, and controllable for the patient and the therapist. Prior to and following any kind of trauma exposition, therapy should focus on establishing psycho-physical stability, discovering and strengthening resources, and establishing safety within the patient's life situation. Patients' individuality must be considered when choosing, forming, and performing interventions.

Traditionally, movement sequences in DMP take longer; have greater amplitude and a higher intensity of dynamics than everyday movements. In trauma-adapted therapy with patients with complex PTSD, however, we must often use what I call "homeopathic doses" of movement, since a tiny portion is sometimes enough to evoke a strong resonance that may frighten the patient. To prevent re-traumatisation, we must recognise and respect the patient's individual level of tolerance. This principle of small steps, which is based on the methodological principles of Luise Reddemann (2006), will be evident in some of the following vignettes.

Moving towards secure attachment

Interpersonal trauma has a destructive effect on the attachment behaviour of survivors (Schore, 2014), compromising the development of affect regulation and self-efficacy. In interaction with the therapist, relational patterns emerge, and attachment ruptured by trauma may be repaired (Wöller, 2013). To this end, nonverbal kinaesthetic empathy and reciprocal interaction are employed, suitable also for attachment trauma suffered in preverbal phases of development, as illustrated in the following vignette.

> Ms Ray came from a family involved in ritual abuse in the third generation. She was very submissive and waited for me to take the lead during therapy sessions. She often laughed nervously, giving me the impression that she was uncomfortable. I began to pause and ask what she felt when she laughed. Ms Ray was surprised that her behaviour had an influence on me. She recognised that she laughed when she felt things were getting too much for her. Upon that, each time she laughed I stopped and asked if something was overwhelming her. On one occasion she said it felt good to have me decipher and respond to her laugh appropriately. I suggested we transform this interaction into a movement activity, the stop-and-go dance. I lead a movement, which Ms Ray could stop whenever she wished. I assured her that I was more interested in respecting her limits than in executing my movement ideas. At her go signal, I began the movement again. In the reflection afterwards, Ms Ray said she would like to try raising her hand in a stop signal, instead of laughing, if she felt overwhelmed. "It's worth my while to give a sign, because you respond to my signals," she said.
>
> In later sessions, we engaged in reciprocal leading/following-stopping. Ms Ray discovered that her fear of initiative was a fear of rejection. She grew to tolerate the limits set by a partner without taking it personally or diminishing her creative energy.

Traumatic experience shapes post-traumatic thought and behaviour patterns of survivors into *trauma compensatory schemas*, consisting of three facets: 1) the aetiological aspect: beliefs about the cause of the traumatic event; 2) the preventative aspect: beliefs about the prevention of such an event in the future; 3) the curative aspect: beliefs about what could heal trauma (Fischer & Riedesser, 2009). Ms Ray believed that being insubordinate by taking initiative or saying no was the cause of abuse. She believed that submissive behaviour was the key to avoiding future abuse. Her ability to assert her limits or ask for help in her overwhelmed state was not totally lost but disguised in a laugh, less likely to provoke the displeasure of a disinclined partner. Sander and Schedlich's (2012) Laban movement analysis study of trauma patients found that trauma compensatory schemas embed themselves into the movement repertoire of a person, causing them to avoid certain movement qualities and emphasise others. For example, many affected persons preferred lightness and avoided strong movement, in order not to draw attention to themselves or provoke anger in others, like Ms Ray's behaviour. In a circular process of interaction with the social environment, this movement repertoire may provoke social partners to complement it, for example responding to a meek quality with a dominant one and reinforce the patient's post-traumatic worldview.

As Ms Ray's therapist, however, I exercised the qualities of "maternal sensitivity" as defined by attachment theory, as a model for therapist behaviour. This *sensitivity* encompasses the ability to: a) perceive signals; b) interpret them correctly; and then respond, c) promptly; and d) appropriately (Grossmann & Grossmann, 2005). In terms of DMP theory, this example shows what *kinaesthetic empathy (KE)* (Sandel, 1993) means; not just mirroring, which in this case would mean I would have joined in the nervous laugh. Instead, the intention of KE is to pick up the emotional core of the expression – in this case discomfort and the wish for a limit – and offer a possibility for regulation, here through stopping and developing a more direct stop signal. Ms Ray revealed later in therapy that her curative belief was that she needed to be seen to heal. This matched well with the intervention of KE.

Rather than remain on the level of minimal interaction with subtle cues (laughing/pausing speech) I aimed to involve the *whole body* in the experience of the pattern of contingent response in the stop-and-go dance. This brings the key interaction sequence *disruption and repair* (Beebe & Lachmann, 1994) to the centre stage of awareness, rather than hidden in the wings, and makes the message "your signals matter" unmistakable. Infant research shows that trust is built not through constant harmony in interaction, but through *repeated mutual repairs* of disrupted interactions through re-attunement, as a primal form of resilience (Shai & Fonagy, 2013). Psychotherapy research shows that outcomes of therapeutic alliances with a rupture-repair pattern tend to be more effective than no-rupture alliances (Larsson, Falkenström, Andersson, & Holmqvist, 2018). The stop-and-go dance becomes a prototype of self-efficacy in relating, which can be referred to in future interactions.

While attachment is vital, so is the development of autonomy and self-regulation through reciprocal interaction (Pickler & Reyna, 2009), to prepare for the termination of therapy. Furthermore, the therapist must practice the purposeful limitation and continuous awareness of the degree of kinaesthetic empathy she employs, to maintain the cognitive, emotional, and physical distinction necessary to facilitate the therapeutic process, and to offer a positive role model for limit setting (MacDonald, 2006).

Deconstructing and reconstructing touch through movement analysis

The importance of touch for the development of attachment is well documented (Duhn, 2010). Often, traumatised patients are brought up with little experience of nurturing, loving touch. Instead, no touch, inappropriate, ambivalent or violent touch (Sbiglio, 2006) characterises interactions. Internalisation processes may lead to patients practicing inappropriate, ambivalent, violent or lack of touch towards themselves and others (Gaensbauer, 2014). Dysfunctional self-touch also entrenches negative self-images of the body as worthless, soiled, incapable, etc. (Schenk & Schedlich, 2001). The question as to when to use touch is one of individual timing. Some patients do not dare to suggest that they wish to work with touch, others with a trauma compensatory pattern of lack of boundaries will suggest touching inappropriately early in therapy. Neither touch-taboos nor forced intimacy effect recovery (Sander & Schedlich, 2007). Instead, therapy should mindfully address self-touch as well as interpersonal touch, to facilitate regulation and to transform thoughts on the meaning of touch. Tantia (2012) suggests beginning with a focus on the environment, such as touching the walls and furniture, going next to activities emphasising the body boundary, and ending with interoception. Accordingly, interpersonal touch may begin with a functional intention, and later an emotional intention may be explored.

Movement analysis deconstructs any type of movement into its components, offering concepts and a vocabulary for diverse qualities. Regarding touch, this enables patients to better recognise inappropriate touch, expand possibilities of regulation, and assimilate new beneficial experiences. Movement analysis correlates movement with cognitive, emotional, and social processes in a developmental framework (Kestenberg-Amighi, Loman & Sossin 2018), used for decoding and encoding meaning. The criteria suggested in Figure 8.1 refer to any situation, not only to therapy, preparing the patient for dealing with situations in everyday life. They can also be used to define ethical therapeutic use of touch.

First, we will consider the social qualities proposed by Anders and Weddemar (2002). *Social context* means the situation in which the touch takes place, such as public (e.g. in a bus), private (e.g. hugging a friend, applying body lotion to oneself), occupational (e.g. at the workplace) or service/medicinal (e.g. in a spa or a physiotherapist's practice). *Intention* refers to the goal of the person doing the touching: is it instrumental, such as supporting a stumbling person, or is it relational, such as stroking someone to express affection or hitting someone to punish them, or professional such as a facial? Intention also makes us aware that some seemingly instrumental touch has a hidden relational intention, such as when someone brushes past while moving down the aisle in a bus, with more surface area than necessary, to arouse themselves. The *determination* of the touch refers to the degree to which the giver and the receiver have influence on the quality and quantity of touch being used. *Safety/trust* considers how well the recipient knows the person touching or whether the role of the toucher gives reason to trust or mistrust them.

Kestenberg-Amighi, Loman and Sossin (2018) offer precise definitions of movement qualities for touch. *Tension flow attributes* encompass three aspects: *intensity*, (also considered by Anders and Weddemar), means the degree of weight invested in the touch, to increase or lessen pressure, evoking qualities such as vehemence or gentleness; *fluctuation* describes whether movement qualities are continuously even or fluctuate; and *temporality* entails the duration of touch and whether it occurs gradually or abruptly, quickly or slowly. *Tension flow rhythm* refers to tension changes in the movement,

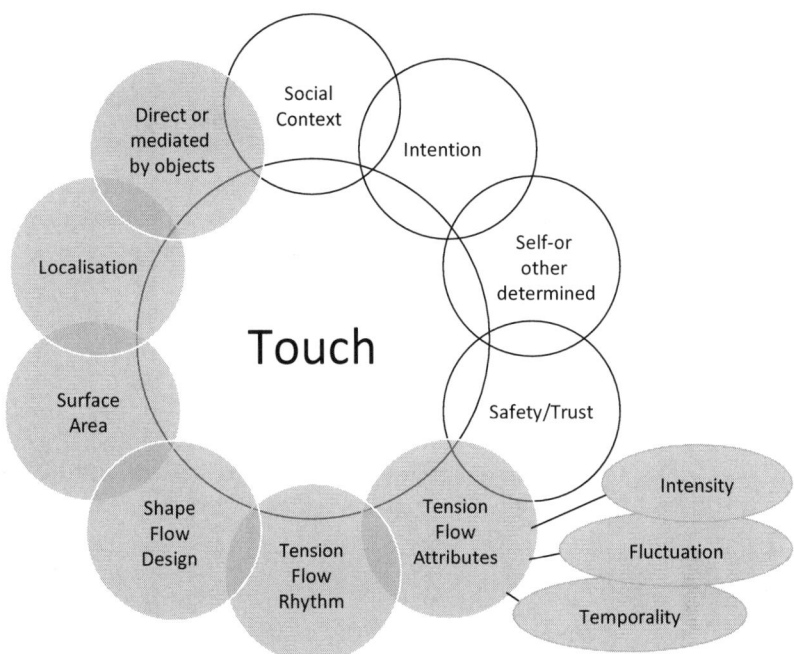

Figure 8.1 Social qualities (white circles) and movement qualities (grey circles) of inter-personal touch.
Expanded from Anders and Weddemar (2001) with additions from Kestenberg-Amighi, Loman & Sossin (2018).

which create various rhythmic qualities such as patting, stroking, twisting, pushing, hitting etc. Circular or straight, even jagged movements during touch constitute the *shape flow design*.

Based on clinical experience I propose *surface area* to refer to the amount of the body which is touched, be it just one spot, or the whole body. Anders and Weddemar (2002) note that *localisation* draws our attention to the body part being touched, and that touch may be *direct*, skin to clothed body or skin to skin, or it may be *mediated by objects*, such as a tennis ball massage or brushing hair with a brush.

The following vignette gives an example of how various qualities come to bear in a process of self-acceptance.

> Mrs Daniels' parents died in a car accident and she was taken into the custody of her aunt and uncle. They made it clear that she was a burden and did not belong. Beatings and sexual abuse followed, and the only way Mrs Daniels could buy her way into the family was to be at the service of others, never resting for a moment.

During a warm-up exercise to support interpersonal boundaries through tension flow rhythms of self-patting various body parts (localisation), Mrs Daniels used inappropriately high intensity, so that the patting was in fact slapping. I showed her how to regulate her intensity and she found a degree that defined her boundaries without being self-abusive. To support boundary setting and safety, we experimented with punting a ball back to the thrower (mediation through an object). Then, using the same quick, brief movement with medium-high intensity, our hands met, and we pushed each other away. She remarked that the even repetition of the same quality (tension flow attribute fluctuation) gave her confidence in me as a reliable partner (safety/trust).

Mrs Daniels brought several drawings expressing her slave-like existence in childhood and in her present family to the next session. A massive exhaustion came over her, and she wished to lie down and rest. I offered her a mat, but as she lay on her stomach she was uneasy and convinced that I disliked such "laziness." I felt the impulse to touch her back and calm her, and told her my idea. Mrs Daniels said with surprise that she'd had the same idea but hadn't dared to speak it aloud. We then negotiated the exact form of touch that would be calming. I demonstrated variations and she chose what fitted (self-determined). It should be between the shoulder blades (location) and not move from there (surface area). The pressure should be of medium intensity: not so light that she thought I wanted to leave, not so strong that it felt like suppression. We agreed that the duration would be one piece of music, three minutes, long. She was able to breathe deeply and rest for the three minutes. Afterwards, I asked Mrs Daniels what she felt the intention of the touch had been. "It said: 'You are welcome to rest.' In fact, 'You are welcome to exist.'" she answered. The following week she noted in her journal three occasions where resting was difficult, but by activating the body memory of the welcoming hand she experienced a welcoming attitude towards herself.

This example demonstrates an important methodological consideration: to stabilise boundaries through fighting qualities, before modalities that encourage yielding are implemented. Feeling confident about being able to set limits makes it possible to explore closeness and gentle touch.

Reclaiming dissociated fragments through metaphor

In the process of dissociation, a person under the extreme stress of trauma may involuntarily separate their thoughts or imaginations from their body sensations to survive. In the case of repeated traumatisation, dissociation becomes a voluntarily induced technique of self-protection, which in chronic cases becomes a seemingly irreversible loss of contact with the body (Young, 1992). However, our brain-body-environment system is programmed to constantly produce associations. Through the neurological co-activation of motor, affective, and cognitive areas of the brain, body-based image schemas develop that can be metaphorically projected to structure our abstract reasoning in ongoing problematic situations (Johnson, 2007).

For example, the repeated association of emotional sadness with the sensory-motor experiences of the downwards motion of the body, through the loss of muscular tension and the falling of tears, activate the image schema of *verti-cality* across various domains of experience. This is then projected onto the metaphor "emotional sadness is a downward motion." This process is reflected in our speech: we understand the statement "I'm feeling down" semantically, and on a sensory-motor level. Various sensory stimuli with a downward ten-dency, such as falling leaves in autumn (visual), successively deepening musical notes (acoustic), the pull of a heavy bag on our shoulder (haptic) etc., can trigger the association of sadness anew. This is one reason why seemingly meaningless stimuli trigger flashbacks. It is also a way of reconnecting split-off affects and physical sensations. Movements involving downward motions may access sadness, such as sinking with the body, lowering a scarf, or dropping flower petals (Eberhard-Kaechele, 2012).

In the following example, a patient had stored the image schema of verti-cality as a substance running down her legs and associated this image to three different events.

> A patient with unexplained diarrhoea showed a constant cramped smile. The hospital staff considered the possibility that grief might be involved in both symptoms, but the patient insisted that there was no cause for grief in her history. During individual DMT she agreed to explore her smile in movement. With large scarves we created a movement metaphor for smiling, holding them up high, wide, and taut. Then we created the opposite, letting the scarf sink limply, narrowly, downwards. Repeating these movements, the patient recognised that "smiling" protected her behind the scarf, while the yet unnamed other state left her exposed. Repeatedly, she let the scarf sink a little further, until she finally let it fall completely down her legs. Then she suddenly remembered having been forced by her mother to have an abortion as a teenager. Her furious mother did not accompany her, and she had walked home alone from the "angel maker" with blood streaming down her legs, as the scarf had just done, as her symptom of diarrhoea did.

The clinical vignette illustrates the phenomenon of emergence, when patterns evolve out of undifferentiated movement elements, generating new meaning.

Creative transformation of post-traumatic representations of self and others

Fischer and Riedesser (2009) argue that the major impact of abuse and neglect in complex trauma is on a person's internal representations of self and other, inferred from how she or he was treated by caretakers. These representations persist as implicit working models rather than as conscious thought. As Briere (2002, p. 176) notes:

> This notion of internalized models or schemas emphasizes the structural or organizing aspects of this phenomenon, as opposed to the presence of discrete cognitions or episodic memories. These core beliefs and assumptions are often relatively nonresponsive to superficial verbal reassurance or the expressed alternate views of others later in life, since they are not, in fact, verbally-mediated.

The choreographic process of *training, improvisation, composition, performance, and reflection* is an opportunity to externalise inner models or schemas, and experience sensory input to challenge their validity. While *training* expands the patient's behaviour repertoire, creative *improvisation* develops problem solving abilities, like stress inoculation techniques (Meichenbaum, 2007). *Composition* formulates a cohesive narrative from fragmented sensory impressions on an abstract or symbolic level that may counteract dissociative tendencies, by creating a safe distance to traumatic experience. The choreographic process empowers the individual with control over the depicted situation, potentially transforming the inner meanings of events, and allowing for the discovery and practice of alternative coping strategies (Sander & Schedlich, 2007). Such self-efficacy experiences are vital for changing trauma-induced negative self-judgements (van der Kolk, 2015). These concepts are illustrated in the following vignette.

> Lilly entered in-patient treatment after having been beaten repeatedly by her husband. She was convinced that she was guilty of something and had somehow deserved this abuse. During a dance improvisation, Lilly was playfully captured by a couple who joined hands on either side of her. She froze and turned deathly pale, giving her captors a fright. After reorienting herself in the present through sensory stimuli (handling and describing various small balls), Lilly remarked that she had a flashback to a key experience from her childhood. Weeks later she expressed the wish to get a grasp on what she felt was the key to her illness and recovery. The group DMP setting seemed most appropriate to her, as Lilly needed witnesses to validate and contain her story.
>
> Lilly explained that her parents were addicted to drugs and alcohol and she was given to foster parents as an infant, after severe neglect. When Lilly reached school age her parents fought to have her returned to them, to cash in on child care benefits. In a move to sway the welfare service they bought Lilly a dog she named Rusty. Lilly's father told her, the dog was not to disturb his peace, and she did all she could to train him to be quiet, so grateful to have a companion and a source of comfort. In the scene that represented Lilly's experience of living with her parents, Rusty had barked

suddenly, which Lilly was not able to prevent. Her father drew a gun out of a drawer and shot the animal before her eyes. All she felt was endless guilt, that she had not saved Rusty's life.

Lilly composed the scene by having group members stand in a circle as the walls of the apartment and the legal custody in which she was trapped with the neglectful, violent parents. They were to face inward and watch if Lilly was okay, but if she was in trouble and wanted out, they should turn their backs. It became clear to her, that this circle also represented the social environment of relatives, neighbours, and child welfare workers who looked away, not seeming to see or respond to her plight.

Within the circle was the intoxicated, demanding mother figure, the lively dog figure, the father figure, erratically aiming a gun at varying targets, and the Lilly figure, running back and forth between caring for the mother and the dog, until she froze at the gunshot. Once movement roles had been assigned the group performed the piece, with the intention of acknowledging the predicament Lilly faced as a child. The group members gave their all, and there were intense emotions to be seen and felt. To her surprise, no one expressed Lilly's primary emotion of guilt. Instead they showed fear of being next in line to be killed, anger at the father for killing the puppy, at the mother for not stopping him, and at the social environment for not rescuing her. And they felt awe at Lilly's survival instinct.

In the reflection, Lilly recognised that the figures in the choreography were parts of her present life. Rusty was her vitality that had been squelched, she had become an alcoholic like her mother, and she had married a violent man like her father. She was trapped in her marriage and in an exploitative job, like she had been in the parents' apartment. Lilly requested a second act, in which she could join the choreography and take responsibility for change. Before it began, I clarified that the second act applied to the present, not the past, for we cannot change the past, only the patterns we learned from it. Now Lilly refused to bring her "mother" alcohol, she linked arms with her vitality embodied by Rusty and left the circle, then called the police to deal with her father/husband.

Experiences stored in implicit, emotional memory must be activated on a perceptual level, by means of sensorimotor stimuli, to be reprocessed (van der Kolk, 2015). Through the intense emotions expressed by the group and activated in Lilly, as well as the concrete sensory interactions in movement, her inner representations were challenged and new impulses for transformation were awakened.

Conclusion

The aspects highlighted in this chapter are only a few of the possibilities of DMP to address the sequelae of complex trauma, which lie beyond words. To do justice to the challenges faced by patients, it is essential to understand why words are not enough for the treatment of interpersonal trauma, and to base interventions on these grounds. Then the sensory, symbolic, and creative techniques provided in arts therapies like DMP can most effectively complement verbal and biological approaches in the interdisciplinary treatment process required by trauma survivors.

References

Anders, W. & Weddemar, S. (2002). *Häute sch(ö)n berührt? Körperkontakt in Entwicklung und Erziehung.* Dortmund, Germany: Bojmann.

Beebe, B. & Lachmann, F. M. (1994). Representation and internalization in infancy: Three principles of salience. *Psychoanalytical Psychology* 11(2), 127–165.

Bernstein, B. (1995). Dancing beyond trauma: Women survivors of sexual abuse. In F. Levy (Ed.), *Dance and other expressive therapies* (pp. 41–58). London: Routledge.

Briere, J. (2002). Treating adult survivors of severe childhood abuse and neglect: Further development of an integrative model. In J. Myers, L. Berliner, J. Briere, C. Hendrix, T. Reid, & C. Jenny (Eds.), *The APSAC handbook on child maltreatment*, (2nd edn., pp. 175–203). Newbury Park, CA: Sage.

Duhn, L. (2010). The importance of touch in the development of attachment. *Advances in Neonatal Care*, 10(6), 294–300. doi:10.1097/ANC.0b013e3181fd2263.

Eberhard-Kaechele, M. (2012). Memory, metaphor, and mirroring in movement therapy with trauma patients. In S. Koch, T. Fuchs, M. Summa, & C. Müller, *Body Memory, Metaphor and Movement* (pp. 267–287). Amsterdam, Netherlands: John Benjamins.

Fischer, G. & Riedesser, P. (2009). *Lehrbuch der Psychotraumatologie.* München, Germany: Ernst Reinhardt.

Gaensbauer, T. J. (2014). Embodied simulation, mirror neurons, and the reenactment of trauma in early childhood. *Neuropsychoanalysis*, 13(1), 91–107. doi:10.1080/15294145.2011.10773665.

Grossmann, K. & Grossmann, K. (2005). *Bindungen – das Gefüge psychischer Sicherheit* (2nd edn.). Stuttgart, Germany: Klett-Cotta.

Herman, J. (1992). *Trauma and recovery. The aftermath of violence – from domestic abuse to political terror.* New York: Basic Books.

Johnson, M. (2007). *The meaning of the body. Aesthetics of human understanding.* Chicago, IL: The University of Chicago Press.

Kestenberg-Amighi, J., Loman, S., & Sossin, K. (2018). *The meaning of movement. Embodied developmental, clinical, and cultural perspectives of the Kestenberg Movement Profile.* New York: Routledge.

Larsson, M. H., Falkenström, F., Andersson, G., & Holmqvist, R. (2018). Alliance ruptures and repairs in psychotherapy in primary care. *Psychotherapy Research*, 28(1), 123–136. doi:10.1080/10503307.2016.1174345.

Levy, F. (2005). *Dance/Movement therapy – A healing art* (3rd edn.). Reston, VA: The American Alliance for Health, Physical Education, Recreation and Dance.

MacDonald, J. (2006). Dancing with demons. Dance movement therapy and complex post-traumatic stress disorder. In H. Payne (Ed.), *Dance movement therapy. Theory, Research and practice* (pp. 49–70). London: Routledge.

Meichenbaum, D. (2007). Stress inoculation training: A preventative and treatment approach. In P. Lehrer, R. Woolfolk, & W. Sime (Eds.), *Principles and practice of stress management* (pp. 497–517). New York: Guilford Press.

Pickler, R. & Reyna, A. (2009). Mother-infant synchrony. *Journal of Obstetric, Gynecologic and Neonatal Nursing*, 38(4), 470–477. doi:10.1111/j.1552-6909.2009.01044.x.

Reddemann, L. (2006) *Eine Reise von 1000 Meilen beginnt mit dem ersten Schritt*. Freiburg, Germany: Herder.

Rothschild, B. (2002). *The body remembers – The psychophysiology of trauma and trauma treatment*. New York: W.W. Norton.

Sandel, S. (1993). The process of empathetic reflection in dance therapy. In S. Sandel, S. Chaiklin, & A. Lohn (Eds.), *Foundations of dance/movement therapy. The life and work of Marian Chace* (pp. 98–111). Columbia, SC: American Dance Therapy Association.

Sander, E. & Schedlich, C. (2007). Trauma-adaptierte Tanz- und Ausdruckstherapie. In S. Trautmann-Voigt & B. Voigt (Eds.), *Körper und Kunst in der Psychotraumatologie* (pp. 223–242). Stuttgart, Germany: Schattauer.

Sander, E. & Schedlich, C. (2012). Aspekte der Bewegungsanalyse und Trauma. Repräsentanz traumakompensatorischer Aspekte im Bewegungsverhalten komplex traumatisierter Frauen. *Zeitschrift für Tanztherapie* 34, 5–13.

Sbiglio, M. G. (2006). Dance/movement therapy and nonverbal assessment of family violence. A pilot comparative study. In S. C. Koch & I. Bräuninger (Eds.), *Advances in dance/movement therapy* (pp. 142–153). Berlin, Germany: Logos.

Schenk, B. & Schedlich, C. (2001). Trauma und Körperbild. In S. Trautmann-Voigt & B. Voigt, *Bewegung und Bedeutung* (pp. 102–111). Köln, Germany: Claus Richter.

Schore, A. (2014). Dysregulation of the right brain: A fundamental mechanism of traumatic attachment and the psychopathogenesis of PTSD. In G. Leo (Ed.), *Neuroscience and psychoanalysis* (pp. 197–235). Lecce, Italy: Frenis Zero.

Shai, D. & Fonagy, P. (2013). Beyond words: Parental embodied mentalizing and the parent-infant dance. In M. Mikulincer & P. Shaver (Eds.), *Mechanisms of social connection: From brain to group* (pp. 185–203). Washington, DC: American Psychological Association.

Tantia, J. F. (2012). Mindfulness and dance/movement therapy for treating trauma. In L. Rappaport (Ed.), *Mindfulness in the creative arts therapies* (pp. 96–107). London: Jessica Kingsley.

van der Kolk, B. (2015). *The body keeps the score: Brain, mind, and body in the healing of trauma*. New York: Penguin Random House.

Wöller, W. (2013). *Trauma und Persönlichkeitsstörungen* (2nd edn.). Stuttgart, Germany: Schattauer.

Young, L. (1992). Sexual abuse and the problem of embodiment. *Child Abuse & Neglect*, 42(1), pp. 89–100.

Chapter 9

The warrior's journey

Linda Winn

The foundation for TMOC

Individuals who have experienced a traumatic event often find that it precipitates a crisis. It can feel that their whole world has turned upside down. This disruption may adversely affect their ability to function in daily life. This is a normal response and after a while the acute distress often subsides. However, for some individuals the crisis causes them to seek psychological help. When addressing the crisis it is helpful to think about what may be maintaining the state. Kfir (1989) identified "the components of crisis" as:

- lack of information
- lack of support
- lack of options

The trajectory of crisis is illuminated in the work of an anthropologist, Victor Turner (1967/1975). His doctoral studies and subsequent lifelong work involved the study of the Ndembu tribe in Zambia This contributed to him creating the Four Phase Theory of Crisis. Turner's observations of the stages of crisis built on the Rites de Passage identified by the ethnographer Van Gennep (1960). Van Gennep identified the three stages marked by ritual as: separation, liminality, and incorporation. The term liminal comes from the Latin, limen, meaning at the threshold, the term used to denote the base of a doorway, which needs to be crossed to enter a building (Harris, 2009; Jennings, 1987; Turner, 1967/1975).

Turner frequently describes liminality as "betwixt and between" (Turner, 1975). He sees it as a temporal state, something people transition through, to a new state of being. This is framed by his studies of ritual. The liminal space allows resting, reflection, and restoration, leading to transformation (Winn, 1998, 2016). Conversely, being "betwixt and between" can leave people feeling stuck or in limbo. This is often the experience of the client that seeks help.

I adapted the use of TMOC for dramatherapy incorporating the components of crisis (Winn, 1998).

TMOC allows a distancing from the heat of psychological trauma. Factors that influence the response to the traumatic experience can be examined. Positive elements that can be harnessed and negative factors that may maintain a reverberating crisis response can be identified and discussed. It assists the therapist to bring clarity into the session. It is a collaborative way of working, which can contribute to the client feeling empowered and in control. This is of importance when working with clients suffering from trauma. Often they will be focused on the feelings of disempowerment that occurred during the traumatic incident (Herman, 2015). TMOC provides a way to discover resources and use a problem-solving approach. This enables a path to be explored in the search for a way forwards in life. In my research, individuals reported that having a visual representation helped them in the therapy space. It also assisted them in recollecting or recreating TMOC for themselves afterwards (Winn, 1998, 2016).

The paper-based TMOC

The client is asked to draw their own TMOC.

Schechner (2003) illustrates a simple linear form of Turner's Four Phase Theory of Crisis. Many clients draw something similar, others spontaneously elaborate by drawing stick people, or placing objects, such as buttons or collage pieces, and using string on their illustration.

The *breach* is an area of fragility for the client (Jennings, personal communication, April 5, 2016). For example, the breach could be developmental; have arisen from an earlier traumatic experience or be related to an attachment difficulty (Pearlman and Courtois, 2005; D'andrea, Ford, Stolbach, Spinazzola, & van der Kolk, 2012). Some individuals would have had a similar experience but have developed resilience from the experience (Bensimon, 2012; Lahad & Leykin, 2015). Others might not be aware of their vulnerability until they have felt challenged by a traumatic incident. It is important to give the client space to express what they see as the breach. It is not necessary to identify a breach if one is not forthcoming. Later on, the client may reflect on the process and suggest a breach that makes sense to them. The *precipitating event* might be a major traumatic experience but could also be a relatively minor trauma in the client's life, but be enough to tip the scale in terms of the cumulative effect of traumatic experiences. The *crisis* ensues, as they attempt to gain equilibrium (*redressive action*). At this stage of discussion of the client's diagram, the therapist can use the "components of crisis" (Kfir, 1989) to identify negative factors, which maintain the crisis, and positive factors that may provide clues to a way forwards. The client may speak metaphorically or may provide concrete examples. Either way, it becomes a problem-solving approach. Initially the client may only identify one positive possibility. This may be built on over several sessions. I find it quite common for a client to return for the next session having identified further positive factors that will assist them to move towards reintegration or separation. Reintegration can be into a renewed "self" or back into a social structure. The client may identify separation as necessary if a cultural or social situation is proving detrimental to recovery.

The paper-based model is useful as an assessment tool and, later on, to review progress or explore why someone appears "stuck." I do not use TMOC in the first session to allow time for some trust to develop between us. In the case of someone who is affected by psychological trauma, a sense of a "safe space" should be established as an initial priority (Gersie, 1991; Lahad & Doron, 2010; Redfern, 2014; Winn 1998, 2016).

The diagram of TMOC is helpful preparation for a "walkthrough" at a later stage. It is also beneficial if the person's level of disability precludes much, if any, physical movement. If the therapist has limited physical space the use of a drawing allows for exploration within the theatre of the mind. As illustrated in the examples from practice (see p. 107), people experience physiological responses and travel through their journey even while outwardly remaining in the same place.

The process of the paper-based TMOC

A brief example of how the TMOC diagram can be used is given before the client commences their TMOC. Care must be taken that the example does not contain elements that will influence the person's own story or be related to their traumatic experience. Examples I have used have been from a play, a current television programme or film that is known to the person (Winn, 1998). An explanation of the components that might lead to a crisis should also be given. As with any therapeutic intervention, the client must be assured that they can stop at any time and reminded of their safe space. The safe space is an area in the room that the client identifies and knows they can move to at any time. Consideration should be given to a client who is unable to move, to identify with them how they will signal the need to enter their safe space, within their mind's eye, or through use of a particular object or signal (Lahad & Doron, 2010; Redfern, 2014; Winn, 1994). They are then given a piece of paper to draw their diagram on. I usually use A4 paper as this helps to maintain the drawing within the field of vision. Some people choose to work on their drawing alone. Others like to discuss possibilities, particularly in the identification of positive and negative factors. It is common for some elements to feature in both the positive and negative columns. It can be useful to prompt the person to identify how they may have dealt with the situation in the past (Winn, 2016). A person suffering from trauma may have become disconnected from who they were before the trauma. They have made it through the trauma or they would not be in the room now (Levine, 1997; Rothschild, 2003). Reframing gently by providing this information can assist the client to consider a new angle.

Practice examples

The examples are from anonimised transcripts from my PhD research with combat veterans (Winn, 2016)

Alan

As Alan commenced his TMOC diagram I enquired whether his military training could help him to plan his journey, he responded: *"The important thing is I pick the route, where I want to go, no one tells me, I decide whether I want to go"* *[chuckles]*.

He described how he was shaking at the start of the session *"but now [inhales deeply] can I just look at you* [sic] *and say I feel in control. I can pick the path."*

The shaking Alan referred to at the commencement of the session related to an intense memory of an incident. The muscle group affected replicated an embodied memory from that traumatic recall (Levine, 1997). His release of the energy resulted in his changed posture and interaction displayed by his deep inhalation, deliberate eye contact and assertion that *"I feel in control. I can pick the path."* The change suggested a turning point (Redfern, 2014; Winn, 2016). He was physiologically and verbally displaying readiness for moving forwards. It was a rebuttal to the fact that he had felt unprepared at the commencement of the session. Although the TMOC drawing session may seem a passive method for dramatherapy, the body is very much part of the action (Lahad, Farhi, Leykin, & Kaplansky, 2010; Levine, 1997; Rothschild, 2003).

Jack

During his TMOC diagram Jack illustrated his ambivalence about who he is since his accident, he described being at war with himself. He viewed himself as having two parts:

> It does feel like that – I've said before in metaphors about Batman – I always wanted to be the Batman, to go forth – it [the character of Batman] wants to encourage me to help others and it wants to keep reminding me where I belong and what your true colours are.
>
> It comes from feeling weak, that you want just to be left alone, and the isolation, it's like the flight thing, you feel like shutting yourself in, you feel unbelievably weak, but it goes from one spectrum to the complete other – one minute it's bend your knees, bend your knees, your body won't work, you just can't take it any longer hearing someone making a noise or fighting, then all of a sudden, it flips over to anger.
>
> I go from complete terror and fear to weak. I find the flight response, it only goes so far then it hits in, it hits in, and goes "No – that way." Then it's fight, fight.

Jack described succinctly how he experienced PTSD. His TMOC drawing provided a focus for him. He identified the dilemmas that are obstacles to his progress on his journey towards reintegration. The identification of the obstacles on his pathway gave him a sense of purpose. He summed up what he wants to achieve.

> I do, I want to win, in a bizarre way, it's not really a competition, but I want to learn how to beat all this other stuff and once I've cracked it and worked out how to do it I want to help other veterans, with housing and everything else. I want to be able to use that information properly.

The "walkthrough" TMOC

Individual TMOC

Explanations should be given at the beginning of the session as part of the warm-up. It is important to ascertain that the client is willing to participate in the journey. I offer either a basic example of a TMOC sculpt or a photographic example. Basic safety guidance is given to pre-empt the possibility of an unstable high-rise structure being made for climbing! The walkthrough is often completed within 30 minutes but time should be made for reflection afterwards and to avoid cutting short the client's exploration.

To prepare for the "walkthrough" (a term given by the research participants) TMOC, the person is first asked to identify and mark out a safe space within the room that they can withdraw to at any time.

A 3D model (sculpt) is created by the client from long cloths and props available in the room to create a pathway that can be journeyed through. They are invited to comment briefly on their sculpt as they begin to move through it. The role for the therapist is to witness and if requested, accompany the person on their journey through the model. If the client becomes stuck, you can enquire what you might do to assist. There is a subtle change to the relationship; the client has the opportunity to become the director of the scene. The client will often want to revisit parts of the TMOC or walk through the whole model several times. You can ask whether they want a photograph of their construction for future reference. The client is reminded to de-role the objects used as they dismantle their sculpt. The client and anyone else involved in the TMOC are also assisted to de-role.

Group TMOC

Sometimes TMOC is used within a group setting. The preparatory phase remains the same and an assurance of confidentiality between group members is sought. The individual still creates their personal walk. The other group members become the audience. They witness the performance and they might be invited by the client to act parts. It is made clear this is by agreement and only if requested. The group members should already be part of an established group. No one is compelled to share a TMOC within the session. The de-roling and reflective period takes place after each TMOC.

Practice examples

Alan

Alan commented on the warm-up phase as I directed the group in moving slowly around the room, paying attention to their breathing and how their bodies felt.

> Alan: If this was a long journey, like that, I could do this for days.
> Me: Right, so you've got your pace?
> Alan: Yeh, I'm into it. I've got my pace, it's dead slow, I don't usually do that, it's easy, and the journey can last as long as it takes now.

Alan would have been used to pacing himself when he was in the military, for marches that may last days. In his anxiety-driven, post-trauma state, he had forgotten the sense of control within that could be found in slow deliberate movement. As he embodied this movement he prepared for the possibility of other roles.

During his TMOC walkthrough with me Alan replicated an abstract battle scene. This evoked strong emotion and while instructing me to *"hold the ground"* he retreated to his safe space. Taking a deep breath, he returned to the scene and instructed me to *"stand down,"* stating that *"we have been victorious and the battle is won."* There was a sense that it had been an internal battle as well as a re-creation of a memory. There was a change in Alan physically as well as mentally at this turning point. He walked in a purposeful upright manner to his destination but then said he wanted to go back to the start and walk through the nice [transformed in his mind] parts.

> Right. I have a vision here of the nice rocks and nice sea, that's good. The insecurity down there [gesturing down the model] has gone.

His eyes watered; this time he said it was with happiness. He rehearsed the scene again, building on the positive images, sights, sounds, and smells.

At the end of his "walkthrough" Alan turned to the other veterans who had been witnessing the scene and exclaimed:

> You've got to have a go of this [sic]. It's not difficult. It's just what comes into your mind. ... Honestly, it's really good. I was just travelling and thinking what on earth is happening here. And it's changed.

Therapist reflections

Outlined above is a brief selection from Alan's TMOC, overall, his "walk-through" took about 45 minutes. As the therapist, I was aware of the need to give him time to decide what he wanted to do and how he would construct his journey. I entered into the space and it was transformed for me. It was a similar experience to becoming involved in a play. At times the experience was vivid and as I was invited to mirror Alan's movements, I was aware of the tension within my body and a change in my level of alertness. It gave me a brief glimpse and thoughts of how it must be to hold that tension within muscle memory and the mind for many years. I have emphasised the need to build client trust; there is also a need as the therapist to trust the client as well as the process. When I was instructed to "hold the ground" I did so with a sense of strength and confidence. It would not have been the time to waiver. I was reminded of the importance of keeping one part of me, as the observer in the room, off-stage (Glass, 2006; Landy, 1996). My clinical self remained available, if required, for Alan or the other group members. I needed to de-role as much as Alan. Supervision provided further opportunity to explore transference and counter-transference (Jones & Dokter, 2008; Lahad, 2000; Wilson & Lindy, 1994).

Jack

Jack referred back to the previous sessions and the work we had been doing on an adaptation of *The Odyssey* (Armitage, 2008) He had found it difficult to countenance Odysseus returning from battle as an old man. Now, as he moved through his TMOC, he stood tall and projected his voice loud and clear, inhaling deeply.

> Now I feel like I'm 35 with the common sense and wisdom of an older man and I've still got my strength – I'm still strong, fit and fast and this is not the end of a dream ...
>
> (Jack)

He had embodied the positive traits he saw in the older Odysseus and took this forward with him as he cleared obstacles out of his way. Sometimes the physical constraints caused by his disabilities made Jack feel aged. He experienced a turning point, equating ageing with wisdom.

As Jack walked through his TMOC he visibly altered his stance as he progressed. Initially he requested that I accompany him, about halfway through, he said I was *"now safe and can step out of the pathway."* He was upright, confident, and speaking with conviction as he reached his destination. He looked back at the model he had just walked through as he stood at his destination: *"but what I thought it's more of an epiphany for me."* He gestured to the area that represented the negative military experiences.

No – no that's great, they're gone now, it's where I'm gonna go now and it's open – it's blank, it's like Highway 9 – I don't know what's coming. But unlike being there, where I knew nothing, as my military told me, I was useless, these voices are so far behind now that I can go past all this, I remember it – bad, bad, bad, bad, bad, bad, bad – but now I'm here – there, that's where I'm going (pointing forward) that's my journey.

He was standing upright and firm *"eyes front."* He had been transformed from the start of his journey through TMOC. He addressed us and emphasised the "bad" loudly, with feeling. He was excited not intimidated by the prospect of a "blank canvas." A sense of a turning point was palpable.

Therapist reflections

The beginning of Jack's "walkthrough" had been intense. As I accompanied him on his journey I became more aware of his hopes and confidence as he progressed in his military career. Initially I was mirroring him but then on his direction became the person he rescued. This was when he received life-changing injuries. It felt to me that I was abruptly dismissed from the scene. However, for Jack, it was the first time he had verbalised the reality, he had saved someone's life. I no longer needed to be in the action as I was "safe." As I stepped to the side as directed, I left the role of injured person behind. I was then off-stage in the role of witness with the other audience/group members. We listened as Jack re-scripted his narrative. The role of audience as witness endorses his story. Theoretically I am aware of how trauma manifests in the body, however to observe the physical change in Jack as he referred to his "epiphany" was moving. He was often quick to anger but now that had been replaced by hope and joy.

TMOC and reflections – thoughts from research

The above examples were taken from my PhD research into veterans' perspectives on the use of dramatherapy to treat psychological trauma (Winn, 2016). The research used mixed methods: qualitative evaluation and quantitative measures (Creswell, J. W. & Creswell, J. D. 2017). Applying Smith, Flowers, and Larkin's (2009) Interpretative Phenomenological Analysis (IPA) enabled me to explore in depth, the content and process of the recorded sessions and capture the veterans' perceptions on TMOC. The veterans elected to film their "walkthroughs."

TMOC used distancing as participants created their own journey through crisis (Turner, 1975; Winn, 1994; Winn, 1998). The physical journey through the model gave the opportunity to use movement to provide greater flexibility in distancing and to move to a "safe place" if wished.

Imagery and Metaphor

The use of imagery and metaphor within the dramatherapy sessions often occurred spontaneously as the participants searched for ways to express their journeys. It allowed them to voice the unspeakable, expressing what is often beyond ordinary language. The language of metaphor proved a useful contribution for finding a pathway through traumatic memories (Jones, 2007; Lahad, 1995; Morris, 2014; Turner, 1975).

Reflections on the use of TMOC with the veterans.

Alan and Jack's perceptions were that they found the use of TMOC beneficial. However, preparation and pacing are important in providing a foundation for TMOC. The risk of re-traumatisation needs to be considered and managed (Chu, 2011). Introducing the use of the model through working with a diagram can assist in preparation for the "walkthrough." The combined use of TMOC (Schechner, 2003; Turner, 1986 with the Components of Crisis (Kfir, 1989) *gave the opportunity for problem solving and assessment of current strengths and deficits.* The creation of the physical TMOC and moving through it emphasises the journeying process. For the veterans, the physical movement appears to have been a key to unlocking muscle memory that helped them recall how they had coped with challenge when in military service. The effect of muscle memory and the role it can have on maintaining traumatic reactions is a consideration in treating PTSD (Rothschild, 2003; van der Kolk, McFarlane, & Weisaeth, 2012).

Alan and Jack described TMOC as "the most useful intervention" they had experienced during their years in therapy. However, distancing methods require caution because of the ability to go deeper into the psyche. This was highlighted by a reflection from Alan following his initial experience with his TMOC diagram. The physical movement in the "walkthrough" appeared to have mitigated this. It may be that the movement, as opposed to sitting in a chair, gave the option of being in control of the scene. This concurs with the acknowledgement of the usefulness of bodywork in the release of trauma (Jennings, 1987; van der Kolk, McFarlane, and Weisaeth, 2012; Levine, 1997; Rothschild, 2003).

TMOC enabled both veterans to experience turning points in their personal journey. The structure of the model provided a safe container, as identified by Gersie (1991). Through the rehearsal of past strengths and problem-solving skills, instilled or built on during military service, they moved forwards through their TMOC sculpt. The distancing through TMOC meant they were not overwhelmed. Instead they countered the physical and psychological stress response by the rehearsal of reprised and alternative roles. As they travelled through the TMOC a liminal space may have been encountered (Harris, 2009; Jennings, 1995; Turner, 1967). At that stage they were able to exercise the *what if* of the imagination and come up with alternative strategies to continue on their journey (Lahad & Doron, 2010). The invocation of this resulted in the veterans' declarations of turning points.

The use of distancing enhances the possibilities of the transformation as was discovered by the participants. The paper-based, chair-bound TMOC provided an opportunity to experience the model, to practise and discuss it. It provided a further method of assessment as the participants identified positive factors that helped them and the negative factors that kept them within a reverberating spiral of crisis.

TMOC training and supervision

I have emphasised the need for building resources and a "safe place" before encouraging others to embark on their journey through TMOC. Working within competencies is a prerequisite for practice for psychological therapists. There are times that clients may be encouraged to step out of their comfort zone but someone suffering from the effects of trauma has probably had more than their share of unpredictability. They need to feel an assurance that the therapist is able to contain what might emerge during the session and between sessions (Gersie & King, 1990; Sajnani & Johnson, 2014; Winn, 1994, 1998, 2016).

I recommend TMOC be experienced by the therapist in a workshop or with colleagues. It is not necessary, and in a workshop not apt, to choose a traumatic episode for the journeying process. Instead, for example, the story of becoming a therapist could be used.

Frequent clinical supervision is an imperative when working with trauma to reduce the risk of vicarious traumatisation (Chesner & Zografou, 2013; Jones & Dokter, 2008; Lahad, 2000; Sajnani & Johnson, 2014). The diagram model and the "walkthrough" can both be used in clinical supervision. The supervisee is able to convey their perspective on therapy or other work-related situation. Alternative strategies can be considered and explored further with the client/s. In my own supervision and reflective practice, I find the opportunity to use TMOC to review a situation helpful. This is particularly so, when the therapeutic process feels stuck. The paradox is that the distancing provided through TMOC can bring clarity to the situation.

References

Armitage, S. (2008). *The Odyssey*. New York: W.W. Norton.

Bensimon, M. (2012). Elaboration on the association between trauma, PTSD and post-traumatic growth: The role of trait resilience. *Personality and Individual Differences*, 52(7), 782–787. doi:10.1016/j.paid.2012.01.011.

Chesner, A. & Zografou, L. (2013). *Creative supervision across modalities: Theory and applications for therapists, counsellors and other helping professionals*. London: Jessica Kingsley.

Chu, J. (2011). *Rebuilding shattered lives* (2nd edn.). New Jersey, NJ: Wiley.

Creswell, J. W. & Creswell, J. D. (2017). *Research design: Qualitative, quantitative, and mixed methods approaches.* London: Sage.

D'andrea, W., Ford, J., Stolbach, B., Spinazzola, J., & van der Kolk, B. A. (2012). Understanding interpersonal trauma in children: Why we need a developmentally appropriate trauma diagnosis. *American Journal of Orthopsychiatry*, 82(2), 187.

Gersie, A. (1991). *Storymaking in bereavement.* London: Jessica Kingsley.

Gersie, A. & King, N. (1990). *Storymaking in education and therapy.* London: Jessica Kingsley.

Glass, J. (2006). Working Toward Aesthetic Distance. In Lois Carey (Ed.), (p. 57), *Expressive and creative arts methods for trauma survivors.* London: Jessica Kingsley.

Harris, D. (2009). The paradox of expressing speechless terror: Ritual liminality in the creative arts therapies' treatment of posttraumatic distress. *The Arts In Psychotherapy*, 36(2), 94–104. doi:10.1016/j.aip.2009.01.006.

Herman, J. (2015). *Trauma and recovery: The aftermath of violence—from domestic abuse to political terror.* New York: Basic Books.

Jennings, S. (1995). *Theatre, ritual and transformation: the Senoi Temiars* (1st edn.). London: Routledge.

Jennings, S. (1987). Dramatherapy: Symbolic structure symbolic process. *Dramatherapy*, 10(2), 3–7. doi:10.1080/02630672.1987.9689319.

Jennings, S. (2016). EPR with adults. Personal communication [e-mail 4 May].

Jones, P. (2007). *Drama as therapy* (2nd edn.). London: Routledge.

Jones, P. & Dokter, D. (2008). *Supervision of dramatherapy.* London: Routledge.

Kfir, N. (1989). *Crisis intervention verbatim* (pp. 15, 21, 23). London: Taylor & Francis.

Lahad, M. (1995). Masking the gas mask: Brief intervention using metaphor, imagery, movement and enactment. In A. Gersie, *Dramatic approaches to brief therapy.* (pp. 139–145). London: Jessica Kingsley.

Lahad, M. (2000). *Creative supervision: The use of expressive arts methods in supervision and self-supervision.* London: Jessica Kingsley.

Lahad, M. & Doron, M. (2010). Protocol for treatment of post traumatic stress disorder: SEE FAR CBT model. *Beyond Cognitive Behavior Therapy* (Vol. 70). IOS press.

Lahad, M., Farhi, M., Leykin, D., & Kaplansky, N. (2010). Preliminary study of a new integrative approach in treating post-traumatic stress disorder: SEE FAR CBT. *The Arts in Psychotherapy*, 37(5), 391–399. doi:10.1016/j.aip.2010.07.003.

Lahad, M. & Leykin, D. (2015). The integrative model of resiliency: The "BASIC Ph" model, or what do we know about survival? Retrieved from www.icspc.org/wp-content/uploads/articles/The-Integrative-Model-Of-Resiliency-The-BASIC-Ph-Model-Or-What-Do-We-Know-About-Survival.pdf.

Landy, R. J. (1996). Drama therapy and distancing: Reflections on theory and clinical application. *The Arts in Psychotherapy*, 23(5), 367–373. doi:10.1016/s0197-4556(96)00052-4.

Levine, P. (1997). *Waking the tiger: Healing trauma – The innate capacity to transform overwhelming experience* (1st edn.). California: North Atlantic Books.

Morris, N. (2014). Silenced in childhood: A survivor of abuse finds her voice through group dramatherapy. *Dramatherapy*, 36(1), 3–17. doi:10.1080/02630672.2014.926958.

Pearlman, L. A. & Courtois, C. A. (2005). Clinical applications of the attachment framework: Relational treatment of complex trauma. *Journal of Traumatic Stress: Official Publication of The International Society for Traumatic Stress Studies*, 18(5), 449–459.

Redfern, M. (2014). Safe spaces and scary encounters: Core therapeutic elements of trauma-informed dramatherapy. In D. Read Johnson & N. Sajnani, *Trauma informed drama therapy: Transforming clinics, classrooms, and communities* (1st edn., pp. 365–388.). Springfield, IL: Charles C. Thomas.

Rothschild, B. (2003). *The body remembers casebook* (1st edn.). New York, NY: W.W. Norton.

Sajnani, N. & Johnson, D. (2014). *Trauma-informed drama therapy.* Springfield, IL: Charles C. Thomas.

Schechner, R. (2003). *Performance theory.* (2nd edn., p. 213). New York: Routledge.

Smith, J., Flowers, P., & Larkin, M. (2009). *Interpretative phenomenological analysis.* London: Sage.

Turner, V. (1967). *The forest of symbols* (1st edn.). New York: Cornell University Press.

Turner, V. (1974). *Dramas, fields, and metaphors.* New York: Cornell University Press.

Turner, V. (1986). *The anthropology of performance.* New York: PAJ Publications.

van der Kolk, B. A., McFarlane, A. C., & Weisaeth, L. (Eds.). (2012). *Traumatic stress: The effects of overwhelming experience on mind, body, and society.* London: Guilford Press.

Van Gennep, A. (1960). *The rites of passage* (1st edn.). Chicago, IL: Univ. of Chicago Press.

Wilson, J. P. & Lindy, J. D. (Eds.) (1994), *Countertransference in the Treatment of PTSD.* New York: Guilford Press.

Winn, L. C. (1994). *Post-traumatic stress disorder and dramatherapy.* London: Jessica Kingsley.

Winn, L. C. (1998). Towards a model of dramatherapy for the assessment and treatment of PTSD (MPhil). Exeter University.

Winn, L. C. (2016). *Combat veterans' perspectives on a dramatherapy journey: A phenomenological mixed methods case study* (Doctoral dissertation, Anglia Ruskin University). Retrieved from https://arro.anglia.ac.uk/702160/.

Chapter 10

Letting go of the spider

Aileen Webber and Sophia Condaris

This case study describes the individual integrative arts psychotherapy work undertaken by a young woman called Celeste. The work took place in private practice over a two-year period. Key identifying elements have been changed to protect the client's identity. Many details have been omitted – including the inevitable impasses that form part of the therapeutic work. The case study and its subsequent analysis are the work of two therapists (the authors) who, for the sake of clarity and readability, are presented as one.

Integrative arts psychotherapy

In the co-created goals made at the beginning of our work together, my client Celeste found it difficult to put into words what she wanted from a therapeutic intervention. She had referred herself for therapy because she felt overwhelmed by powerful, unmanageable feelings that were affecting her daily life. She had tried a purely verbal psychotherapy but had not found it useful, ironically sitting in silence for most of the time. She was an art student and experienced the visual arts as enjoyable and cathartic, and so she referred herself to me. My practice offers integrative arts psychotherapy – a multi-modal, arts-based approach in which the therapist provides a variety of integrated arts media to support each client's own unique therapeutic work (Knill, Levine & Levine, 2005). It is also integrative in that it combines a number of theories across the psychodynamic, humanistic, and behavioural schools (Evans & Gilbert, 2005); acknowledging that clients need both verbal and non-verbal ways of working.

The unspeakable

I wondered for weeks if Celeste would be able to tell me the source of her anguish. She wept through most of our first sessions. Her breathing was shallow, her voice a whisper, and she spoke only haltingly. There were periods of silence that seemed full of affective charge, but it was difficult to connect with her because she would simply stare at the floor. My words of empathy had little visible effect. The only thing that appeared to emotionally regulate her was creating images with the art materials available in my practice room. She made abstract paintings of vivid, swirling colour, which she would then dramatically defile with black crayon or splatter over with black paint. But she could not tell me what had brought her to therapy.

In addition to art materials, the practice room contains shelves of sand-tray figures and miniatures. At the beginning of her sixth session, Celeste selected a wooden bear cub from these shelves. She held it closely and appeared to be soothed by stroking it. Soon after, she returned and selected a larger bear. She placed the two bears together on the rug. She went back and chose as many mother and baby pairings as she could find until the centre of the rug was crowded: a gorilla and its baby, a raffia doll and its miniature, a big snake and a little snake, a Russian *Matryoshka* doll, and the smallest doll from its nest. Finally, she selected a large piece of black fabric and draped it over all the figures.

Although her weeping continued, Celeste appeared somewhat calmed by having created this image. We sat in silence allowing the power of what she had made to impact us. I considered saying something but my words felt inadequate to meet her raw grief and desolation. Instead, I selected a single flower from the shelves and placed it ceremonially in front of the shrouded figures, as though laying flowers on a grave. I began to sing softly a song of grief with a simple melody. I repeated the refrain several times and Celeste, hesitatingly at first, began to sing along. When the song came to an end, Celeste said through her tears that she had recently received the devastating diagnosis of infertility, at age twenty-six.

Enter the spider

In our next session Celeste was more animated and verbal. She surprised me when she came into the room and started recounting a dream not obviously connected to her image from the previous week:

> I am in bed asleep. I wake up because I become aware there is something on my back. I try to shrug it away. It's massive and heavy and stuck to my skin. I try to scream but no sound comes out. I realise it's a tattoo of a huge spider that is coming alive … I can feel its legs clawing at me. I try to scream again. In the dream, I think: "it's trying to eat me." Then I wake up.

I suggested she create an image inspired by the dream. She chose to use a sand-tray, and carefully selected several eggs and placed them in a circle in the sand. She then selected the figure of a young girl and placed it in the corner. She found some large plastic spiders and, disgusted by them, tipped a heap into the corner of the tray, behind the girl. I thought they looked like an army, ready to attack. She placed one of these spiders on the girl's back. Finally, she took a heap of minuscule spiders and placed them at the centre of the circle of eggs.

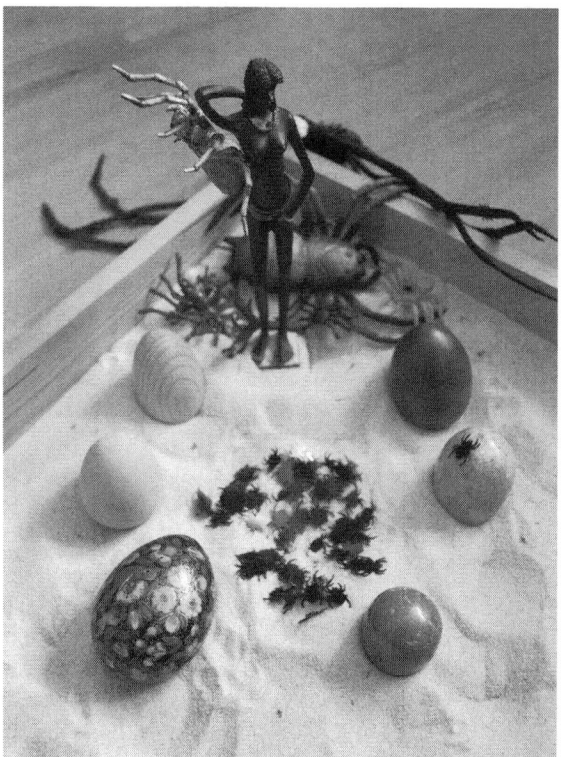

Figure 10.1 Spider sand tray

What happened next caused us both to gasp. As she reached into the sand-tray to adjust one of its elements, one of the smaller spiders leapt into the air, seemingly of its own volition, and landed on top of the blue marble egg. "The spider is *eating my eggs*," she exclaimed in horror.

Poetry

Over the following weeks, Celeste began to speak more openly about the impact of her infertility diagnosis. It was clear she was battling existential issues of *meaning* (Yalom, 1980) arising from the issue, and her grief was often anguished and inconsolable. She wrote a series of poems, many of which spoke of her longing:

To my unborn child

If I call you, will you come to me?

With your round honeyed head and your little cry?

If I sing your name again and again

Will you nestle here close to my heartbeat and

Be comforted by it?

If I reach out and stretch further than I ever have before

Will you cross over time and space, lean down with your sweet breath

against my ear and whisper

Here I am, Mummy.

Maman

At the beginning of a later session, Celeste said she had been thinking about spiders. She had started drawing them and looking for representations in art. She told me about Louise Bourgeois' sculptures of spiders (Bourgeois, 1999) and described a "massive" one called *Maman* [*French:* mother]. She showed me several images of Bourgeois', including one in which the arachnid's legs and body encompassed a steel cage where, as Celeste put it, the spider "keeps its prisoners" (Bourgeois, 1997). Sometime later, she felt strongly compelled to make an image of her womb overtaken by a huge spider-crab. When I asked if it had a title, she named it, "*The Body Snatcher.*"

During the next stage of her therapy we explored memories from Celeste's childhood. I thought they might throw light on the mysterious, recurring theme of the devouring spider. She made sand-tray images and drew pictures to depict her childhood family home. I encouraged her to create a timeline of her life (which included dates, drawings, and objects placed upon a scroll of paper stretched across the floor). She was making this timeline when she revealed to me that when she was thirteen her parents separated and her father went to work overseas. Her mother had become extremely ill and struggled to look after Celeste. I noticed her level of anxiety increase as she came to this part of her narrative. I named that she looked scared and reminded her she was safe in the room with me. I suggested she drew something to represent the part of her story she found too difficult to speak about. She used a crayon and drew the childlike outline of a house, teetering on the edge of a cliff. Above it, she wrote the words, "A Year Away from Home." Then she selected a large spider and placed it alongside the house. Here, for the first time in our work, she had given the spider symbolism (Jung, 1952) a specific location and time in her history. She wrote, "The Lost Year" at the bottom of the page and spent a long time looking at the image she had made. I asked permission to sit beside her – to offer additional support but also to see the image from her perspective. I felt strongly affected by it; by the smallness of the house hanging from the cliff-edge, and the relative vastness of the spider.

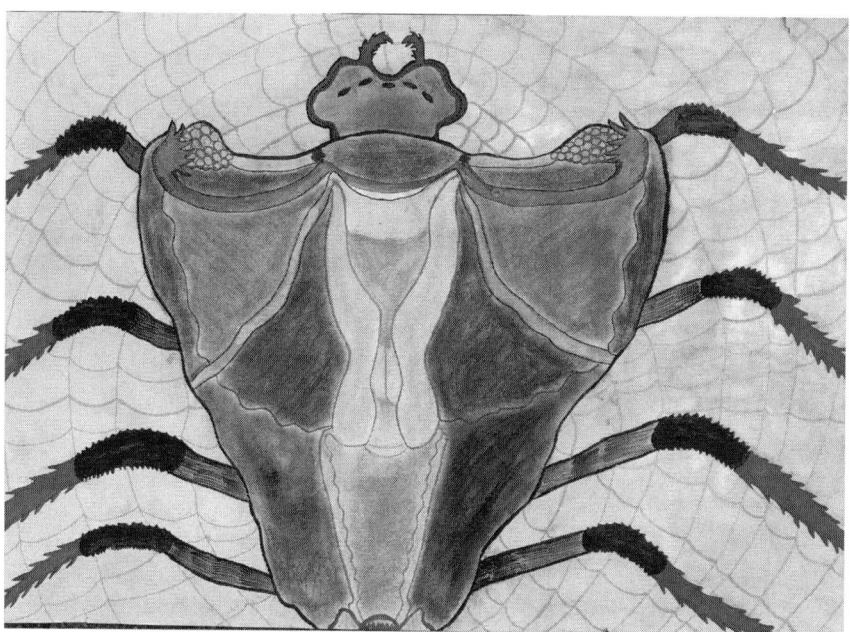

Figure 10.2 Body Snatcher

The lost year

The following week Celeste told me she had been thinking deeply about *The Lost Year*. She found herself tormented by disturbing memories and unsettling feelings from this time. She wanted to continue working on her image from the previous session. She selected the figure of a small girl and placed it in front of the house, facing the giant spider. I spoke directly to this child character. I said I could see she was all alone with a frightening-looking spider. Celeste was able to nod but not able to speak, so I suggested she write a poem from the perspective of the girl. She wrote and then read aloud:

The lost year

You filled me with fear

My life was lost for a year.

Round my feet, your sticky web

Round my hands and neck, tighter and tighter until I was nearly dead

Round my heart and tender places

You told me time and again how odd my face is

You said: "You are ugly and wrong.

You are stupid and your legs are too long

No one will want you when you're grown

You'll have no children and be on your own

Look, you're bleeding, you nasty thing

I know what I'll do – I'll clip your wings."

It was difficult to catch all the words because she sobbed as she read. I did not know the details of what had happened in this house but she had clearly and powerfully communicated the horror of her experience.

The bird in the castle

Celeste often brought paintings and drawings to therapy. They enabled her to uncover hidden feelings and memories concerning *The Lost Year*. For example, she brought in several versions of a shadowy female figure with her mouth taped shut.

When I asked if the gagged woman in Celeste's image had ever spoken aloud, Celeste said she had, "a long time ago, when she felt safe in her home." She went on to make a home out of fabric and cushions, and carefully placed her drawing of the woman inside, where the gagged woman felt safe enough to tell her story:

> Once upon a time, there was a bird who lived inside a crumbling castle. A monster-sized, spider entrapped this bird in its web and would not release her … The Monster Spider was sadistic in many different ways; she would taunt the bird, tie up her wings and say she was ugly. She said cruel things like, "you will never mate or nest or see your fledglings fly." Sometimes the Monster Spider would pretend to let the bird escape and then, at the last minute, spin a new web and catch her again.

Creating and telling this story appeared to unlock something in Celeste and for the first time she felt able to reveal details of her *Lost Year*. She told me she had been sent away to live with her father's aunt when her mother was ill and her father had been working overseas. Her great aunt had been viciously unkind and mercilessly shamed Celeste, at a time when she was a budding adolescent, coping with the seminal experience of her first menstruation and its accompanying bodily changes. Her aunt said she was a "dirty, smelly girl" and forced her to hand-wash her blood-stained sheets. She threatened to hang the soiled sheets outside for all to see if Celeste did not do as she was told. She also made frequently disparaging comments about Celeste's developing breasts, claiming she was too unattractive to ever find a partner.

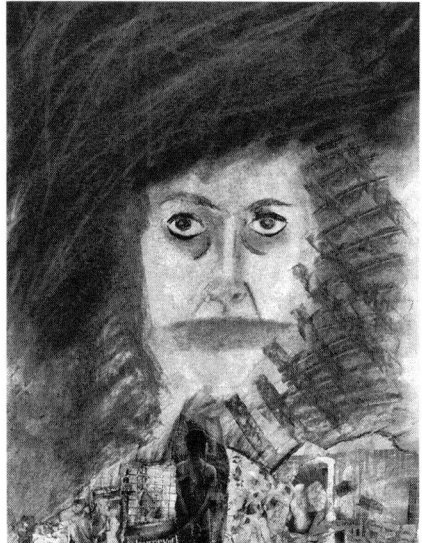

Figure 10.3a Gagged woman 1

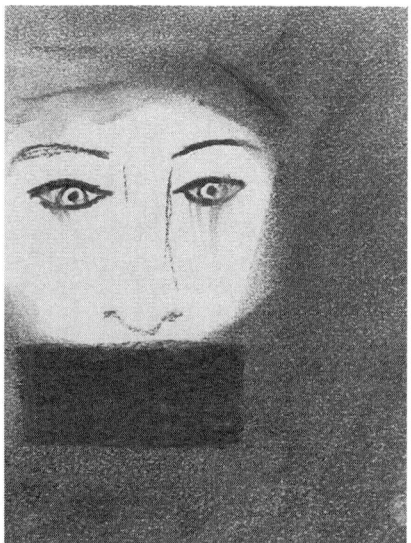

Figure 10.3b Gagged woman 2

When Celeste went back to live with her mother at the end of this year, she decided to tell no one of the cruelty inflicted upon her. It became her secret *Lost Year*. But through months of artistic creation and exploration, she had been able to recover and reveal this time. We were now able to link the experience to her dream of the spider tattoo, her images of the woman gagged, and the house teetering on the cliff-edge. Celeste realised the experience with her aunt had deeply affected her perception of herself as a woman. She considered herself unattractive and plain; she hated her body and menstruating. She also recognised her life choices to date had been linked to the fear she was defective in some way. She began to wonder how much *The Lost Year* had negatively impacted her body, and even perhaps contributed to her infertility.

Celeste also began to connect with her rage about the experience. She created paintings full of explosive energy and colour in her sessions. Outside of therapy she began boxing as an outlet for her anger.

Then, in one session, she made a model of a spider with crumpled newspaper for its body and wool-covered wire for its legs. I noted the spider was now smaller than it had been in previous images. At my suggestion, she explored how she felt when she placed herself and the spider in different places in the room and if there was anything else she wanted to do with the spider. She made a tree with large roots out of clay, to symbolise "the woods." She hollowed out a space for the spider to go inside and placed pieces of fabric, leaves, and paper on top. At the end of the session, she deliberately and ceremoniously turned away from the spider, leaving it behind in the woods.

Letting go of the spider

Sometime later, she relayed a dream from the previous night:

> I am in a new house. I'm pregnant and know the baby is coming soon. I squat down and am horrified to find what comes out is a bloody spidery creature with long legs. I rush to a doctor in another room and tell him what's happened. He's completely unperturbed and wishes me well. I wake up in a cold sweat.

I suggested she speak first as herself in the dream. She communicated strong revulsion on seeing the grotesque collapsed spider come out of her womb. I then asked if the doctor could share his perspective. The doctor said the Monster Spider had taken up residence inside Celeste for a long time. He affirmed Celeste in undertaking the difficult work of expelling *Maman* and deactivating the power of her great aunt. The link between this role-play and the "spider-crab womb" image she had previously created, astonished Celeste and left us both marvelling at the remarkable power of the arts and the human psyche.

Reflections on the work

Integrated theories

As an integrative practitioner, I drew from a broad range of sources and wove them together to understand Celeste's therapy. These were based on what I believe it means to be human, how difficulties may arise, and also from my experience of being in the room with Celeste. I found insights from neuroscience invaluable in identifying the impact on Celeste of her traumatic experience.

The psychodynamic tradition, with its emphasis on the impact of childhood experiences and unconscious processes, was central to my understanding of Celeste's therapy. Freud and Jung, and theoreticians from the Object Relations School (e.g. Bateman & Holmes, 1995, Nolan, 2002) contributed to the basis of this work. Psychodynamic principles are based on the premise that past experiences are influential in shaping thoughts, feelings, and behaviours. Ascertaining Celeste's developmental history was difficult as she struggled to verbalise in the initial stages of therapy, and she had also convinced herself that the experiences with her great aunt were not significant. These were repressed and not consciously brought into therapy (Freud, 1961a). Until her dream of the spider (Jung, 1952), she appeared to have no awareness of how intensely the trauma had affected her. Jung saw the unconscious as a great guide and adviser of the conscious, and he believed this guidance often presents itself through symbols and dreams (ibid.).

The degrading treatment by her aunt that had violated Celeste's adolescent body, was felt viscerally in the horror of the spider symbol. Because she had kept her trauma secret she had no idea that the internal *object-relationship* (Nolan, 2002) with her aunt had been exerting an unconscious influence (Freud, 1961b) that had deeply affected her subsequent relationship with herself as a woman, partner, and potential mother. The symbol of the spider enabled her to access memories, and through increasing awareness and understanding unconscious patterns, Celeste was able to slowly rebuild a narrative of what had happened to her.

Also, included in my integrative stance were theoretical ideas from the humanistic tradition: including Perls (1973), Mann (2010), Rothschild (2000), Clarkson (1990), and Kaufman (1991). My way of working usually focuses on the client's experience in the here and now and fits closely with the Gestalt experiential approach (Perls, 1973). Rather than providing interpretation or analysis, the client's awareness is increased by the active use of experimentation (Mann, 2010). However, Celeste had experienced a past trauma, so if we had worked experientially on *The Lost Year* too soon, it could have potentially traumatised her again. Celeste's body remembered her *Lost Year* even though she tried to keep it hidden. As Rothschild explains: "Trauma is a psychophysical experience, even when the traumatic event causes no direct bodily harm" (Rothschild, 2000, p. 5). In the room with me, Celeste's *muscular armour* (Reich, 1945) was visibly communicated through her shallow breathing, tension, trembling, and quiet voice. This *armour* was an attempt to protect her from overwhelming feelings of fear, distress, grief, and recollected helplessness and horror.

Celeste's *Lost Year* and the upsetting emotions associated with that time, were unprocessed and unresolved, known in Gestalt terms as *unfinished business* (Perls, 1973). The traumatic experience became entrenched in a rigidly *fixed Gestalt* (ibid.), creating an unending pattern of fear, intrusion, and avoidance (Mann, 2010). By using symbols and metaphors, we were able to work in the here and now, as it was at a level somewhat removed from the experience that she found too difficult to speak about. In addition, because emotional regulation was very difficult for her, creating images of her experience allowed Celeste to give external form to her internal bodily sensations, and gain some relief from retaining them in her body.

Concepts from Badenoch (2008) and van der Kolk (2015) supplied neuroscientific explanations for how psychotherapy could support Celeste. Synapses in the brain become "woven into neural nets that become isolated baskets holding terror, pain and shame" (Badenoch, 2008, p. xxii). By working through her trauma with multiple arts media, Celeste was able to begin to integrate some of these isolated "neural nets" within her brain and psyche. Research has shown that in the event of a traumatic experience, the Broca's area (one of the brain's language centres) is deactivated (van der Kolk, 2015). Celeste frequently had no access to language and so image making and creative writing were vital in providing her with the means to externalise her internal world and share her experience.

Van der Kolk suggests that "safety and terror are incompatible" and that in order to recover, "mind, body, and brain need to be convinced that it is safe to let go." (van der Kolk, 2015, p. 201). This requires the client to feel able to connect that sense of safety with "memories of past helplessness" (ibid.). In this respect, the relational aspect of Celeste's therapy was a crucial part of creating safety for her. Countertransferentially I felt that the work needed to proceed slowly and carefully. I was aware that any sudden (metaphorical) movements might frighten her; she often seemed like a deer that could easily become startled and run away. It was an enormous challenge for me to keep her in close contact with the material without her withdrawing or becoming traumatised again. At times I felt she was unreachable; partly from the desolation of her grief and her considerable feelings of shame (Kaufman, 1991), but also because her body would respond to traumatic events as though they were happening in the here and now (Perls, 1973).

The therapeutic relationship needed to provide a corrective experience (Clarkson, 1990). As a young girl, the adult that was elected to be Celeste's caregiver, violated her trust in an appalling way, and she subsequently did not feel able to seek out a trusted adult to help her with her considerable distress. The secure, empathic, relational alliance provided by the therapy and the metaphorical work through the arts, enabled her to eventually trust and increase her capacity to regulate her intense feelings. By giving her agency over which aspects of her experience to explore and affirming her capacity to manage within the safety of the relationship, over time Celeste was able to process and integrate *The Lost Year*.

Integrated arts

The therapeutic approach in this case study is grounded in the *interrelatedness* (Knill, et al., 2005) of the arts. By using an assortment of arts media over time, Celeste found herself able to speak about her infertility and reveal her experiences of the year spent with her great aunt. Knill, et al., have observed that each of the different arts media has a unique benefit in assisting therapeutic work. Combining them enables a client to utilise their own preferred expressive style for a particular aspect of their therapy – visual, tactile, auditory or kinaesthetic (ibid.). In addition, deep trauma frequently cannot be fully processed with one "telling" and needs to be visited multiple times (Badenoch, 2008).

Celeste's use of sand-tray and miniatures allowed her disturbing images to be externalised (Schaverien, 1999), where they could be witnessed and gave her much needed distance from the unsettling material.

The song brought sound to her grief, and allowed me to provide empathic attunement at a deeper level than speech (Sacks, 2007).

Her use of poetry enabled her to reach emotions distilled from intense affect into sensory and imagistic words with compressed meaning (Mazza, 2003). It also allowed her to work at a slower pace than speaking, so she could take time and have a sense of agency (Mollon, 1977) over her experience.

Painting and drawing brought Celeste's newly emerging psychic material into pictorial form and allowed for the expression of feelings and memories. Clay provided a sensory material that enabled her to construct a three-dimensional representation of place (Henley, 2002), where she could leave the image of her abuser. Research has shown that the processing of mental imagery and visual stimuli employs almost all the neural pathways (Hass-Cohen, 2008, cited in Webber, 2017).

Celeste's use of drama and story enabled a metaphorical language (Siegelman, 1990) whereby she could fictionalise her traumatic memories, and allowed the hopeful symbol of the bird to emerge (Jung, 1952).

Creating the timeline accessed a more left-brain, narrative approach (Cozolino, 2002), which helped locate Celeste's story in time and place.

There were layers of psychic protection afforded to Celeste from each of the arts approaches she employed. For example, the "gagged woman," telling her fictionalised story, allowed Celeste a multi-layered experience of distance and safety.

Our therapeutic relationship was a triangular one, of image-client-therapist, (Dalley, 1993) and Celeste's art creations were a pivotal part of her restoration process. Even when she was unable to speak or connect with me, she could remain connected to her art, and I could connect to her through the images she made. In this respect, my role often felt like that of midwife to her images (Waller, 1991).

Letting go

During her remaining time in therapy Celeste created paintings around a new theme. In her sessions and at home she began to produce images connected to the bird that had emerged in her story. We carried out several weeks of therapeutic work featuring the symbolism of this bird. Her final image was of an empty woodland scene. I noticed in the top right-hand corner of the picture, a tiny bird flying away.

References

Badenoch, B. (2008). *Being a brain-wise therapist.* New York: W.W. Norton.

Bateman, A. & Holmes, J. (1995). *Introduction to psychoanalysis: Contemporary theory & practice.* London: Routledge.

Bourgeois, L. (1997). *Spider (Cell)* [Steel, tapestry, wood, glass, fabric, rubber, silver, gold, and bone]. Collection the Easton Foundation, New York.

Bourgeois, L. (1999). *Maman* [Steel and marble]. Collection the Easton Foundation, New York.

Clarkson, P. (1990). A multiplicity of psychotherapeutic relationships. *British Journal of Psychotherapy, 7.*

Cozolino, L. (2002). *The neuroscience of psychotherapy.* New York: W.W. Norton.

Dalley, T. (1993). *3 voices of art therapy: Image, client, therapist.* London: Routledge.

Evans, K. R. & Gilbert, M. C. (2005). *An introduction to integrative psychotherapy.* Basingstoke/New York: Palgrave MacMillan.

Freud, S. (1961a). The interpretation of dreams. In J. Strachey (Ed. & Trans.), *The standard edition of the complete psychological works of Sigmund Freud* (Vol. 4 pt. 1, pp. 5–353). London: Hogarth Press. (Original work published in 1900).

Freud, S. (1961b). The ego and the id. In J. Strachey (Ed. & Trans.), *The standard edition of the complete psychological works of Sigmund Freud* (Vol. 19, pp. 3–66). London: Hogarth Press. (Original work published 1923).

Hass-Cohen, N. (Ed.) (2008). *Art therapy and clinical neuroscience.* London: Jessica Kingsley.

Henley, D. (2002). *Clayworks in art therapy: Plying the sacred circle.* London: Jessica Kingsley.

Jung, C. G. (1952). Symbols of transformation (R. F. C. Hull, Trans.). In H. Read, *et al.,* (Series Eds. Trans.), *The collected works of C.G. Jung* (Vol. 5). Princeton, NJ: Princeton University Press (Original work published 1911).

Kaufman, G. (1991). *Shame: The power of caring.* Cambridge, MA: Schenkman Books.

Knill, P. J., Levine, E. G., & Levine, S. K. (2005). *Principles and practice of expressive arts therapy.* London: Jessica Kingsley.

Mann, D. (2010). *Gestalt Therapy: 100 key points & techniques.* London: Routledge.

Mazza, N. (2003). *Poetry therapy: Theory and practice.* New York: Bruner-Routledge.

Mollon, P. (1977). *The fragile self.* London: Whirr Publishers.

Nolan, P. (2002). *Object relations and integrative traditions and innovation in theory & practice.* New Jersey, NJ: John Wiley.

Perls. F. (1973). *The Gestalt approach & eye witness to therapy.* New York: US Science & Behaviour Books.

Reich, W. (1945). *Character analysis.* New York: Orgone Institute Press.

Rothschild, B. (2000). *The body remembers.* New York: W.W. Norton.

Sacks, O. (2007). *Musicophilia: Tales of music and the brain.* New York: Random House.

Schaverien, J. (1999). *The revealing image.* London: Jessica Kingsley.

Siegelman, E. Y. (1990). *Metaphor & meaning in psychotherapy.* London/New York: The Guilford Press.

van der Kolk, B. (2015). *The body keeps the score.* London: Penguin.

Waller, D. (1991). *Becoming a profession. The history of art therapy in Britain, 1940–1982.* London: Tavistock/Routledge.

Webber, A. (2017). *Breakthrough moments in psychotherapy.* London: Karnac.

Yalom, I. D. (1980). *Existential psychotherapy.* New York: Basic Books.

Chapter 11

An elemental relationship – nature-based trauma therapy

Hayley Marshall

While developing my outdoor practice, I have been interviewed for a great deal of outdoor psychotherapy research. Much of this has focused on the motivation for psychotherapists to take their clinical work outside. It seems that I, and many of my outdoor colleagues, have had childhood histories where connecting with nature formed an effective way of regulating distress. Natural spaces of various kinds have been sought out as places of solace and refuge, offering relationships that were highly effective in managing the world as it was experienced then. Research has also shown that many clients seeking the natural world for their therapeutic space would also very much identify with this childhood process (Jordan, 2015); and instinctively understand that there is something to be found there that is inherently settling.

In this chapter, I will explore relational aspects of a nature-based trauma therapy, viewed through this regulatory lens – specifically focusing on the enlivening, soothing, and resourcing processes that occur in such a dynamic space. I will illustrate elements of the process with case material, written as amalgams in order to protect client identity.

My therapeutic base

I have been practising as a psychotherapist for twenty-three years, and for the last ten I have been working with clients, supervisees, and trainees, outdoors.

Theoretically, my outdoor work is rooted in relational transactional analysis (Hargaden & Sills, 2002). This, combined with the work of Daniel Stern (2010), movement and body therapies (Brantbjerg 2008; Reeve, 2011), cognitive scientist Wilma Bucci (2008), and ecotherapist Martin Jordan (2015), has formed the basis for my own relational theoretical and methodological frame for outdoor psychotherapy (Jordan & Marshall, 2010; Marshall, 2016a; Marshall, 2016b).

The therapy takes place mainly on the move in a large area of open access land – see Figure 11.1.

This landscape comprises a small nature reserve with ponds; streams and waterfalls; mixed woodland; and wilder moorland on the top of a hill.

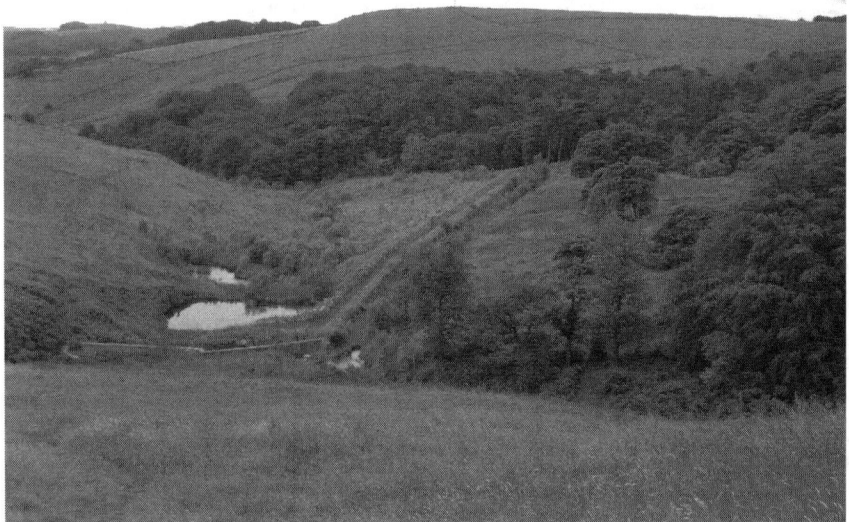

Figure 11.1 Outdoor therapeutic space.

With the natural world acting both as co-therapist and as a fluid, relational context for the therapy, I work with how the client reveals their relational world via the embodied relational process. This involves working with movement, somatic communication, use of space, metaphor, and nature connection, where much of the therapy is in the implicit (non-conscious, nonverbal) realm of experience. However, I also work on an explicit level (conscious, verbal) to develop holding and resourcing in the work.

Relational geography

My new client Nik tells me about her difficulties in relating to others, and that she feels isolated. She mentions briefly that she has experienced some physical abuse by family members. She wants to have her therapy outdoors because she has always been connected to nature since being a very young child. "I felt instantly drawn to this," she says, "I think I will feel safer and need a big space to deal with my past."

Spring

I meet Nik at the small parking area for her first session. We walk up the rough track into the space. As we move I catch her hesitancy in relation to me; although we are side by side she leaves a lot of space between us. She doesn't turn to me at all, keeping her visual focus on the surrounding landscape. She walks so quickly that I am struggling to keep up with her. However, she seems to connect to the place quite readily, commenting on the hills and the vibrant green of the trees. The only time we really stop is for her to pet a passing dog.

I notice her ease in being outside, but I already feel a bit "kept out" by her as she appears to have more of a connection with nature than with me. We have already walked a good way around the nature reserve before Nik begins to talk about what has brought her here. She doesn't say a lot or go into much detail, and I notice I am not saying much either, feeling "silenced" by the process of the walk.

As Nik and I begin to move into the place, I sense her ease in instantly relating to the place, but it feels to me that she is already "inserting" the natural setting between us. She is less settled in her relating with me, appearing to be vigilant about the space between us, and stays physically distant, moving fast, and focusing "out there." This then, is an effective way for her to regulate our contact. She also covers a lot of ground spatially before she gets to why she has come. This can often indicate that the person is literally moving away from contact with their internal experience and contact with me.

My thinking about how space is moved through and related to in this active embodied sense is a development of ideas taken from Daniel Stern's *Forms of Vitality* (2010), and movement practices such as Body and Earth (Olsen, 2002) and Move into Life ™ (Reeve, 2011). In outdoor therapy, I work with how the use of the space reflects the client's relational process (Jordan & Marshall, 2010). This in effect, is the *emotional geography* (Bondi & Fewell, 2003) of the therapy.

So, although Nik doesn't go into detail about her past, I am witnessing important relational information through her physical "interactions" with both me and the natural setting. Even though I do not yet understand the meaning of these, I hold a sense of her difficulty in staying in relationship with human others, and a curiosity about the trauma that may have led to this.

Client-nature-therapist

There are expansive shifts in therapeutic relating outdoors, and one significant element of this altered therapeutic equation is of course, nature – what I term a "living third" (Marshall, 2016a). This "third" is comprised of aspects of the living setting for the work, including animals, trees and plants, water, the weather, and the "space" – the broader landscape itself; all essentially forming a dynamic nonverbal "other" or "others" in the therapeutic relationship. Along with the human to human relating, this provides a rich, fluid, relational dynamic in which client and therapist can discover all kinds of meanings and resources. I understand all of this as a dynamic four-way process, depicted in Figure 11.2.

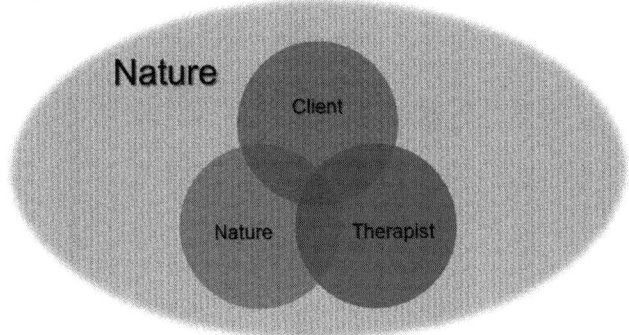

Figure 11.2 Outdoor therapeutic relating (Marshall, 2016b)

This model offers a simple relational structure for outdoor therapy. It illustrates that nature is constantly influencing the human elements all the time – shown by the ellipse – much of this on a non-conscious level. In this way, it offers one of the many containers for the work; but it also forms a more discrete subject in the relational process – shown by a separate circle of its own – flowing in and out of the therapy in more explicit ways. In this sense, both human participants have their own, particular, more conscious relationship with it.

Using this model, it was possible to track where the relational emphases were for Nik, as well as where the work generally needed to be focused. In our relational dynamic Nik situated herself in the overlap between her and nature. She confirmed her strong bond with the natural world had been developed in childhood. She appeared to be managing the human to human in our encounter through a more secure, direct relationship with nature. In working with childhood trauma, I have found that some clients will "use" their relationship with nature as a "protection" from a more direct psychological contact with me. In this – often a transferential process – the client projects elements of people from their past onto me, incorporating nature as a type of relational buffer. In this, nature becomes part of the transferential matrix (Jordan, 2016). In parallel, I understand that the client will also be using this process internally, to help regulate "unbearable" aspects of their traumatic experience.

Nature as a dissociative space

The natural world had been a major resource for Nik at the time of the abuse. She would go to the local woodland near her childhood home to "forget" what was happening to her. Here, she could focus on something else. Nature effectively supported what I understood to be, her dissociative process, in offering her quite literally *a place to escape to*. Therefore, Nik's relationship with a specific place in nature at that time became intertwined with her separated-off thoughts, feelings and body experience relating to the abuse.

I follow many authors (Fisher, 2017; Brothers, 2008), in viewing dissociation as a regulatory, self-restorative process – and concur with van der Kolk (2014), who sees it as "the essence of trauma" (p. 66). Nik's relating with nature in this sense, was a means of maintaining the split in her experience; a way for her to take care of herself at the time of the abuse.

Summer

A few months in and Nik and I walk with her leading the way. Our route has varied little over the weeks following the perimeter of the landscape each time. We climb up to the moor and walk along the top path, coming back down through the trees. She is again moving quite fast, but now has begun to stop a bit more in her sessions to talk. She still doesn't seek very much eye contact, but does turn to me occasionally, indicating changes in the relational process. I'm allowed "in" a bit more.

Today, I decide to comment on how important it seems for her to keep moving; wondering how this affects her experience of me. Looking at the horizon, Nik reflects that she can stay in charge of where I am, making it easier for her to be with me on the move.

Also, looking out to the hills, I say "This seems like a very important way to manage the amount of me you can tolerate then?" She nods.

She then says it's also easier for her if we look out together rather than at each other. "I can begin to stay a bit more in touch with me whilst still knowing you are here."

"These are very smart ways of staying in contact but not getting overwhelmed" I say.

In a session a few weeks later, we come to a halt near a large tree. She leans on one of its thick lower branches and breathes deeply. I wait. She begins to tell me some more about her family. I ask her about the significance of the tree; Nik says "Sorry, but I really do need the support from this."

"Nik, this is you being you. You learnt how to do this a long time ago" I say. "It has been so important to let nature support you like this." Nodding, she moves away from me slightly with tears in her eyes.

In Nik's early therapy we effectively walked around in the world of her dissociation. She appeared unconnected to her experience and to me; continuing to move swiftly around the space with little eye contact, and not that much talking. She engaged with certain trees, animals, and birds encountered along the way, but in a manner that didn't include me in the encounters. Her distance from her trauma experience was being mirrored in her relating with nature; her distance from me; and our physical use of the space. Through moving together, I witnessed and held this implicit (non-conscious and non-verbal) process. In this session, I gently invite her to become more aware of the significance of it –

a gradual coming *alive to the deadening of her dissociation* as it is re-enacted in the natural setting. This was a delicate edge in the work, but my intention was to normalise this self-protective process for Nik.

Relational intensity

This enlivening process involved supporting her awareness of how she was regulating her contact with me. Referring to Figure 11.2, the work centres on the overlap of all three circles between the client, nature, and therapist.

Nik mentioned at the outset that she wanted therapy outside – intuitively understanding that she would feel "safer." Indeed, later on she said that she wouldn't have come for therapy at all if it had been in a room. This highlights a common issue for those who have experienced abuse; that being in an enclosed space with another person is potentially very triggering of the past (Fisher, 2017). This is often coupled with a difficulty concerning managing the human gaze while sitting opposite another. Both of these situations can stimulate the autonomic nervous system into intensified hyper- or hypo-arousal survival states (Brantbjerg, 2015). However, it seems that having therapy outside, especially walking side by side, relieves this intensity somewhat (Jordan, 2015; Brazier, 2018), creating a "window of relational tolerance" to work within.

With Nik, as well as focusing on the physicality of our process, we also work on developing an explicit relationship with the part of her that had creatively connected with nature as a source of support.

This whole way of working is based on Fisher's (2017) use of the structural dissociation model (van der Hart, Nijenhuis & Steele, 2006), and the internal family systems approach (Schwartz, 1995). She outlines a method whereby the work does not necessarily focus on the traumatic events directly, but deals with the client's responses to these events. This is achieved through facilitating the client's present centred connection with the "parts" that helped them survive. Using a transactional analysis lens, I view this as promotion of a dynamic Adult ego states process (Summers, 2011; Marshall, 2016b); how Nik as the adult she is now, begins to understand, accept, and respect the child parts of her that withdrew from other humans, and who reached for nature as a way to survive what was happening to her.

Systemic regulation and natural spaces

Thus far, the work with Nik essentially centres on a key issue in the therapy of trauma – emotional and physiological regulation (Fonagy, Gergely, Jurist, & Target, 2002). There is evidence that nature can provide a unique contribution to this.

It seems that we are predisposed to focus on natural living processes (Wilson, 1993), and these in turn help restore our brain functioning and physiology (Kaplan & Kaplan, 1989; Mind, 2013; Ulrich, 1983), readying us for effective responses to the immediate demands of our environment. There is, therefore, a regulatory implicit fit between us and the natural world.

Environmental psychology research shows that contact with natural environments promotes a *psychophysiological stress reduction response* (Ulrich, 1983) within our limbic system, as well as an activation of an *attentional recovery system* (Kaplan, 1995) in the frontal cortex of our brain. These are ancient survival responses, with the former important for swift recovery from the fight or flight response; and the latter significant in clearing the mind, providing space for reflection and regaining clear cognitive focus.

In outdoor trauma therapy, these restorative and regulatory responses form a significant aspect of the work. The psychophysiological stress reduction response is probably relevant in helping us to regulate affect while in a state of arousal, important when traumatic experiences are surfacing. Alongside this, the attentional recovery response promotes a shift to a more reflective state, thereby assisting the client with the development of verbal sense-making in relation to the trauma experience, named by Bucci (2008) as the referential process.

I understand all these as relational processes forming part of the client's dynamic Adult ego states (Summers, 2011); in that they involve both non-conscious, regulating transactions with the environment, as well as the development of a more conscious Adult ego state process. Referring again to Figure 11.2, we are now dealing with the ellipse, whereby the therapy is infused with nature's vibrancy throughout. It is important to note – apparent from the model – that this regulatory process is also happening for the therapist. Many outdoor therapists report that the natural setting provides significant support for them – particularly relevant when more challenging material surfaces in the countertransference (Jordan, 2015).

While it is clear that there can be nature-promoted self-regulation, true regulation of past trauma, whereby the experience is integrated and assimilated, involves another human nervous system (Brantbjerg, 2015).

Dosing

Consequently, alongside working with Nik's dissociative process I needed to help her move into a more conscious regulatory relationship with me.

Autumn

> Nik and I are walking into the nature reserve. She reports feeling anxious about talking with me today. We move off into a clearing at the side of the track, and spend some time working with her senses as a way of helping to ground her. I then offer her an opportunity to work more directly with the landscape, asking her to notice where in this place she feels can she "tolerate" more or less of me.

Nik takes us down by the bigger of the pools of water, finding it "very calming." She refers to the bowl shape of the land around us, saying "I feel somehow safer down here."

I comment on her "making good choices for her"; and then invite her to place me in the space, at whatever distance from her that feels right. I remind her that she can move too, and suggest she takes time to "dose" this – making any adjustments. She puts me slightly behind one of the small trees, but noticing that this feels like "too little contact," moves me out again. I invite her to tune in to her anxiety levels and any sensations, however small, in her body as a guide. She finally places me a bit closer, with her up above me on a small ledge. From here we talk more about our relationship and how she's feeling about it.

Here we are working more in the territory of the overlap of the therapist and client in Figure 11.2. Nik is taking permission to manage her contact with me more explicitly and therefore, to regulate her experience of anxiety. I invite her to tune into her body in relation to the landscape, noticing what works for her in terms of facilitating contact with me through nuanced adjustments. The aim was to promote Nik's sense of her own inner authority through working with the concept of *dosing* taken from the field of relational trauma therapy (Brantbjerg, 2015). This is a simple but profound principle of resource-oriented skill training, a psychotherapeutic method "that focuses on a sensory based presence here-and-now, and on bridge building between body and language" (Brantbjerg, 2008, p. 5). Working with hypo- and hyper-responsive muscle states in psychomotor exercises, dosing places an emphasis on a client's inner sensing and direction as *the* guide to how much (or how little) is tolerable. Through this process of inner negotiation, a person's presence in the present can be supported, enabling them to maintain contact with themselves and the therapist.

In our process, Nik is supported by me to use her familiar regulatory relationship with nature, and the use of space and distance, but now from an active Adult ego state. Through developing a stronger adult ego state container for her experience, she accesses new resources to regulate triggers relating to the trauma as they arise; as well as developing her capacity to tolerate current experiences (Fisher, 2017).

Containers

To summarise, I understand the work with self and mutual regulatory processes as essentially about helping Nik to access and develop different kinds of "container" to both hold (Winnicott, 1960) and contain (Bion, 1962) her experience. This is an important way of building a sense of safety into the process.

Nature offered a significant containing process for our work. This was present implicitly throughout; but a more explicit example is where the bowl-like form of the landscape itself helped Nik feel safe and held. Her relationship with the space as a whole also seemed important in terms of a holding function, particularly her need to walk the perimeter in the initial sessions. I view this as landscape as "elemental sustenance" (Marshall, 2014; Marshall, 2016b), where aspects of familiar landscapes can offer a holding function "a sense of bringing parts of us together in one physical and psychological place" (Marshall, 2014). Nik also developed attachments to aspects of the landscape providing soothing – e.g. the big beech tree and the pool in the nature reserve.

Alongside this, we were also working more directly with Nik's body as container throughout the work, via movement, sensory work, and some psychomotor resourcing exercises (Brantbjerg & Stepath, 2007). This helped her learn to self-regulate with some new skills and resources, essentially building a containing function whereby her emotional experience could become better tolerated.

The final container was in the development of our relationship – facilitating Nik to tolerate more of my presence within the relational dynamic. A stronger alliance with me would be especially important as some of the implicit trauma fragments surfaced in the process. We could then support her to stay in contact with her trauma experiences while staying grounded – more of a mutual regulatory process.

Through this creation of "a neurobiologically regulating environment" (Fisher, 2017), the aim was that Nik begins to *associate* rather than dissociate, through becoming better resourced in the present. I view this as facilitating the further development of Nik's Adult ego states, to incorporate relationships with nature and the wider landscape; with "parts" that survived the trauma; and with me, all in the present (the overlap of all three circles in Figure 11.2).

Protocol

Although, on one level, nature can be a dissociative space for a client, it is at the same time, an enlivening one. Through a combination of the vitality evident in the place (Jordan, 2015; Marshall 2016b); increased physicality of the process (Marshall, 2016a); and a more expansive relational canvas; a client's dissociated trauma can also be accessed very directly. Offering a heightened sense of immediacy within the process, this obviously needs calibrating – a monitoring of the client's level of arousal (Fisher, 2017). However, with sufficient development of the containers mentioned above, this material can then be worked with so that the client can begin to integrate their trauma.

Winter

> Nik and I set off up the hill through the trees. The weather has turned cold; it is raining hard and the path is very muddy. As we walk Nik begins to slip, and slides into a boggy area off to the side. She tries to lift her feet but her boots are stuck fast. One of them comes off and she steps her foot directly into the mud. Unthinking, instinctively, I laugh. Nik appears to freeze.

I instantly feel appalled by my response. Before I say anything, she frantically reaches for her boot, making to move away from me. Gathering myself, I invite her to slow down and stay with what's happening. She has moved up the hill slightly, putting some distance between us. I stand still.

"I frightened you" I said.

She nods and then leans on a tree nearby as she starts to sob.

"You're OK, just stay with what you're feeling Nik" I say.

"It hurt that you laughed at me" she says, crying.

I pause to let her feel this, and then say "I'm really sorry I did that."

After a while, as Nik becomes more grounded, I suggest we move down to the little bridge across the river in order to help settle her some more before we talk about what has happened. She reports that she felt that the environment became very hostile ... "It's raining, it's muddy ... I was struggling."

She then says that in that moment she'd felt threatened and shamed by me.

"What would have happened next?" I ask. "I would have been beaten up" she says.

Here, Nik contacts part of her trauma experience live in the therapy. I understand this as her accessing an *implicit relational-knowing* (Lyons-Ruth, 1998) from the time of her trauma. Known in transactional analysis as the protocol (Berne, 1972), and described by Cornell as an "incorporation of the environment that the child grows up in" (W. Cornell, personal communication, June 22, 2010); this is a felt sense of "what it was like for me." Protocol is experienced as happening in the present through sensory, somatic, emotional channels. It reflects a sense of "the shape of relating" (Stern, 2010).

With Nik this takes the form of an embodied-relational enactment (Santostefano, 2004), whereby she experiences the "environment" as becoming hostile. The weather is significant, but she also experiences me in that moment as an abusive other. This triggers her trauma response of freezing and wanting to run. I support Nik to stay with her feelings (rather than move away and dissociate), in order to access more of her experience. She also leans on the tree to help her manage her level of overwhelm, going on to tell me what she's feeling – something very new for her. I meet her by owning my part in the process.

Assimilation

As more of Nik's protocol material emerged in our work, she began to feel more present in our relationship. The physical pace of the therapy had slowed right down, and we covered far less of the space in each session. Nik held eye contact more readily, and involved me more, both in her interactions with the environment and with her internal experience. Nik's trauma experience was being – as Cornell and Landaiche (2006, p. 204–205), put it – "brought into awareness, understood and lived within," and thereby opened "to new experience and action."

Spring

As Nik and I sit up on the crag above the reserve, we have a panoramic view over the therapeutic place and to the landscape beyond. We are reviewing our work.

"We have covered a lot of ground together," she says.

She picks out where we've done various pieces of work; where in the landscape she has felt certain things, and accessed particular resources.

She comments that locating these places helps her feel a sense of coherence about what we've been doing; but remembering the location of a connection with certain experiences also helps her hold on to the shift she felt at the time.

She says that it has been important to be "witnessed by this place" as she has done this work.

Conclusion

The significant shifts that occur through introducing nature into the relational matrix bring new ports of entry into a client's trauma states. Nik's therapy illustrates the process of working within the embodied world of her dissociation – strongly associated with nature, while also enlisting this "living third" to breathe new life into her human-to-human relating.

Offering both a stimulating and a soothing environment, nature inherently provides the therapeutic dyad with unique opportunities to reveal elements of past trauma, and also to gain help in regulating anew.

References

Berne, E. (1972). *What do you say after you say hello?*London: Corgi Books.

Bion, W. (1962). *Learning from experience*. London: Karnac Books.

Bondi, L. & Fewell, J. (2003). "Unlocking the cage door": the spatiality of counselling, *Social and Cultural Geography*, 4(4), 527–547.

Brantbjerg, M. H. (2008). Resource-oriented skill training as a psychotherapeutic method. Retrieved from http://moaiku.dk/moaikuenglish/englishlitterature/articles_pdf/a4/ROST_BP_2.2_A4.pdf.

Brantbjerg, M. H. (2015). About survival reactions. In *Relational Trauma Therapy*. Retrieved from http://moaiku.dk/moaikuenglish/englishlitterature/articles_pdf/a4/aboutsurvivalreactions_a4.pdf.

Brantbjerg, M. H. & Stepath, S. (2007). The body as container of instincts, emotions, and feelings. Retrieved from http://moaiku.dk/moaikuenglish/englishlitterature/articles_pdf/a4/TBC_2.0_A4.pdf.

Brazier, C. (2018). *Ecotherapy in practice: A Buddhist model*. Abingdon, UK: Routledge.

Brothers, D. (2008). *Toward a psychology of uncertainty: Trauma-centred psychoanalysis*. New York: Taylor and Francis.

Bucci, W. (2008). The role of bodily experience in emotional organisation: New perspectives on the Multiple Code Theory. In F. Sommer Anderson (Ed.), *Bodies in treatment: The unspoken dimension*. (pp. 51–76). New York: The Analytic Press.

Cornell, W. F. & Landaiche, N. M. (2006). Impasse and intimacy: Applying Berne's concept of script protocol. *Transactional Analysis Journal*, 36(3), 196–213.

Fisher, J. (2017). *Healing the selves of trauma survivors: Overcoming internal self-alienation*. New York: Routledge.

Fonagy, P., Gergely, G., Jurist, E. L., & Target, M. (2002). *Affect regulation, mentalization, and the development of the self*. New York: Other Press.

Hargaden, H. & Sills, C. (2002). *Transactional analysis: A relational perspective*. E. Sussex, UK: Brunner-Routledge.

Jordan, M. (2015). *Nature and therapy*. E. Sussex, UK: Routledge.

Jordan, M. (2016). Ecotherapy as psychotherapy: Towards an ecopsychotherapy. In M. Jordan & J. Hinds (Eds.), *Ecotherapy theory research & practice*. (pp. 58–69). London: Palgrave Macmillan.

Jordan, M. & Marshall, H. (2010). Taking counselling and psychotherapy outside: Destruction or enrichment of the therapeutic frame? *European Journal of Psychotherapy & Counselling*, 12(4), 345–359. doi:10.1080/13642537.2010.530105.

Kaplan, R. & Kaplan, S. (1989). *The experience of nature: A psychological perspective*. Cambridge, UK: Cambridge University Press.

Kaplan, S. (1995). The restorative benefits of nature; toward an integrative framework. *Journal of Environmental Psychology*, 15, 169–182.

Lyons-Ruth, K. (1998). Implicit relational knowing: Its role in development and psychoanalytic treatment. *Infant Mental Health Journal*, 19(3), 282–289.

Marshall, H. (2014). The view from here: A sustaining transaction. *The Transactional Analyst*, 4(3), 40.

Marshall, H. (2016a). A Vital Protocol: working at embodied relational depth in nature-based psychotherapy. In M. Jordan & J. Hinds (Eds.) *Ecotherapy – Theory research & practice* (pp. 148–161). London: Palgrave Macmillan.

Marshall, H. (2016b). Taking therapy outside: Reaching for a vital connection. *Eco-Psychotherapy: Synthesising ecology and psychotherapy in practice and theory*. Retrieved from www.confer.uk.com/module-ecopsychotherapy.html.

Mind. (2013). *Feel better outside, feel better inside: Ecotherapy for mental wellbeing, resilience and recovery*. London: Mind.

Olsen, A. (2002). *Body and earth: An experiential guide*. New Hampshire: UPNE.

Reeve, S. (2011). *Nine ways of seeing a body*. Axminster, UK: Triarchy Press.

Santostefano, S. (2004). *Child therapy in the great outdoors: A relational view*. New Jersey: The Analytic Press.

Schwartz, R. (1995). *Internal family systems therapy*. New York: Guilford Press.

Stern, D. (2010). *Forms of vitality: Exploring dynamic experience in psychology, the arts, psychotherapy, and development*. Oxford: Oxford University Press.

Summers, G. (2011). Dynamic ego states-the significance of nonconscious and unconscious patterns, as well as conscious patterns. In Fowlie, H. & Sills, C. (Eds.). *Relational transactional analysis: Principles in practice*. (pp. 59–67). London: Karnac.

Ulrich, R. (1983). Aesthetic and affective responses to the natural environment. In Altman, I. & Wohlwill, J. F. (Eds.), *Behaviour and the natural environment*. (pp. 85–125). New York: Plerium.

Wilson, E. O. (1993). Biophilia and the conservation ethic. In Kellert, S. R. & Wilson, E. O. (Eds.). *The biophilia hypothesis* (pp. 31–41). Washington DC: Island Press.

Winnicott, D.W. (1960). The theory of the parent-child relationship. *International Journal of psychoanalysis*, 41, 585–595.

van der Kolk, B. (2014). *The body keeps the score: Mind, brain and body in the transformation of trauma*. London: Penguin Books.

van der Hart, O., Nijenhuis, E. R. S., & Steele, K. (2006). *The haunted self: Structural dissociation and the treatment of chronic traumatisation*. New York: W.W. Norton.

Part III

The impact of trauma on the therapist and embodied supervisory approaches

Chapter 12

Secondary traumatisation and therapist illness

Ditty Dokter, Lisa Lea-Weston and Tara Thornewood

Introduction

"Therapists may have a tendency, in a life dedicated to listening intently to others' troubles, to set aside or even ignore their own needs" (North American Dramatherapy Association, 2015). Qualitative systematic review of dramatherapy literature indicated that dramatherapists often provide individual/group therapy to clients who act out their problems through destructive behaviour patterns (Dokter et al., 2011). The stress of containing difficult material can affect the therapist's own mental and physical health, while other life stressors in the therapist's life can exacerbate their vulnerability to this client material. Freud (1905/1997) talks about the effect on the therapist of conjuring the human beast's half-tamed demons. This somewhat melodramatic presentation has worked its way through into the code of ethics of therapists, stressing that therapists need to monitor their own physical, psychological, social, and spiritual well-being to provide clients with the best possible treatment (Johnson & Barnett, 2012).

How well equipped are we as (drama)therapists to recognise whether we absorb too many toxic elements from our work? We may only notice it when we reach burn out, but earlier recognition of secondary trauma or compassion fatigue may provide a useful indicator. There is a professional requirement for regular supervision, which we return to later in this chapter (Jones & Dokter, 2008). Therapists are no more resistant to unexpected or difficult personal circumstances than anyone else (Skovholt & Trotter-Mathison, 2016). Adams (2014) studied the impact of therapists' personal problems such as pain, depression and anxiety, home life as child and adult, illness and death, as well as experiences of violence. She showed therapists' struggles to seek help for themselves and the issues arising in relation to self-care and fitness to practice.

In this chapter, we use our own experience of living with/surviving cancer as a therapist and ask if lessons can be learned from such an experience.

Literature review

Neuroscience and the body in relation to trauma

Trauma is held in the body because it is experienced by the body. The mind does not comprehend it in words. Making the distinction between what is past and present is not possible nor is it possible to see a future. Van der Kolk (2014) asserts that through role play, embodied action, accurate mirroring, a person who has suffered immense trauma can build new neural pathways by enacting a different experience to the one that happened: "physically re-experiencing the past in the present and then reworking it in a safe and supportive 'container' can be powerful enough to create new, supplemental memories." (van der Kolk, 2014, p. 300) As therapists we are constantly attuning to our traumatised clients and work to support their healing in this way. We will experience much of what they are feeling in our own bodies. Since dramatherapy is a body-based therapy, how likely is it that we will also empathically absorb this trauma? It is necessary for effective therapy for us to be able to tune into our clients on each level.

Scaer (2014) investigates the role of traumatic stress in physical symptoms and disease. The premise is that the body reacts to trauma via an evolutionary survival system: fight, flight or freeze responses are triggered by incoming stimuli that are perceived as threatening and interpreted according to past practice. If the system becomes overwhelmed, the body is unable to process these responses and energy cannot be discharged.

There is emergent thinking and recognition that many more people are surviving cancer but that many are left with the symptoms of post-traumatic stress disorder. Much of the writing about trauma and recovery talks about it being in three broad stages, recognised by the authors. The three stages are about safety and stabilisation, remembering traumatic memory, and looking to the future/ reintegration (Rothschild, 2000).

Vicarious traumatisation

Vicarious traumatisation was previously described as professional "burn out" or "compassion fatigue" caused by continuous exposure to others' trauma.

Symptoms of vicarious trauma can include some of the same symptoms as those experienced in the original trauma (Pearlman & McKay, 2008):

- increased fatigue or illness
- social withdrawal
- reduced productivity
- feelings of hopelessness or despair
- work-related nightmares
- feelings of re-experiencing the event

- having unwanted thoughts
- increased sense of danger

Many people come into the healing professions following their own exposure to trauma – the wounded healer (Stevens, 1994). Repeated exposure to others' trauma carries the risk of therapists' own trauma being re-triggered (Levy-Gigi et al., 2015). This risk is acknowledged by the training bodies accredited by the Health and Care Professions Council (HCPC) in the requirements for dramatherapists to undertake personal therapy and clinical supervision during training as well as at points during practice. This ensures that arts therapists pay close attention to any indications of the symptoms of vicarious trauma.

Goleman (1995) writes about the concept of "ready-fire-aim" to describe the negative impact of dissonant, impulse-driven actions in the workplace. Often, traumatised people tend to follow this divergent form of functioning.

In the moment of trauma, we struggle to think. We become stuck in the "fire," the immediate danger. Our brain's amygdala goes into overdrive (i.e. pain, confusion, displacement, fury, disbelief, a burning desire to understand). Not surprisingly, the experience of trauma throws familiar coping mechanisms out of kilter.

The role of the dramatherapist is to be with people who come for help, to redress the balance of the brain's neurons, caught in the crossfire of traumatisation. Stern (1998) refers to the relational mode as a way-of-being-with or style of relating in the context of attachment theory.

Levine (2010) describes his experience of sudden, life-threatening trauma in a road traffic accident. He describes being emotionally held by a female passer-by, in whose presence Levine was able to fully experience the physical shaking of his body, as it struggled to process what had just happened. Levine believes that this was why he did not experience post-traumatic stress.

Impact of therapist illness

A few trials exist assessing the impact of arts therapies on breast cancer patients (Boehm et al., 2014), emphasising the effects on depression, anxiety, and quality of life. A few accounts exist of arts therapists' autobiographical experience of cancer, including artistic exploration (e.g. Wadeson, 2011, CD of art work included in the book; Alker, 2015, with performance). Breast cancer's causes are a mix of environmental, social genetic/family factors, which are different for everyone. One in eight women in the UK have a lifetime chance of developing breast cancer in the UK (www.breastcancercare.org.uk).

How clients are told about their therapist's illness is important. The fact that therapist illness impacts on clients is widely accepted, although under-researched in terms of frequency, how it is worked with by that therapist and other staff, including "foster" parents (Edwards, 2016. The impact on therapists and their ability to practice is more widely publicised (Wilton, 2001). How much detail about therapist illness to share with the client is an interesting area for research (Kaufman, 2016).

Autoethnographic stories

Introduction

The writing style of autoethnography includes realist, confessional, and impressionist tales (van Maanen, 1988). It has been used by arts therapists to research intercultural factors of their background (Mullen-Williams, 2016) and is used here to study the impact of illness experience.

"In using oneself as an ethnographic exemplar, the researcher is freed from the traditional conventions of writing. One's unique voicings – complete with colloquialisms, reverberations from multiple relationships, and emotional expressiveness – is honored" (Gergen & Gergen, 2002, p. 14).

Ditty's story

In spring 2011, I received further investigation after a routine mammogram found abnormalities. I was diagnosed with breast cancer and advised I needed surgery. I was in the first year of a new academic post and head of an NHS arts therapies department, a post I had been active in for several years (see Figure 12.1).

The NHS team and manager were very supportive and advised, with support from the occupational health (OH) department, that I should go on sick leave until the completion of treatment. It was the end of the academic year for the students, and the university manager and team supported me in working from home to complete assessments and to help plan the next academic year. As I was the only established dramatherapy member of staff, extra visiting lecturer staff were appointed to hold the fort while I was off sick for the autumn. The difficulty was that I was in my probationary year, so annual leave was used to cover some of my sickness period. Despite the support and equality legislation I was very aware of my insecure situation regarding my academic employment. My manager ensured that my probationary year appraisal was completed favourably while I was ill, so that no adverse circumstances of my illness would hamper my completion of the year. I felt very fortunate in the support of my colleagues. My clinical supervisors and managers enabled me to take time to process my diagnosis and prepare myself for treatment. I also had time to let family and friends know and garner support for the care of my ageing parents in a different country.

Diagnosis was late May/early June, surgery in July, followed by radiotherapy (August/September) and medication, envisaged for five years started in September. I received good support from what was then the Wallace (now Maggie's) Centre in Cambridge, which provided support during and post treatment for both patients and their carers. It supported me in dealing with side effects of treatment, but also in the recovery stage with yoga, qi gong, nutrition, a women's support group, and coaching to return to work. Despite the excellent

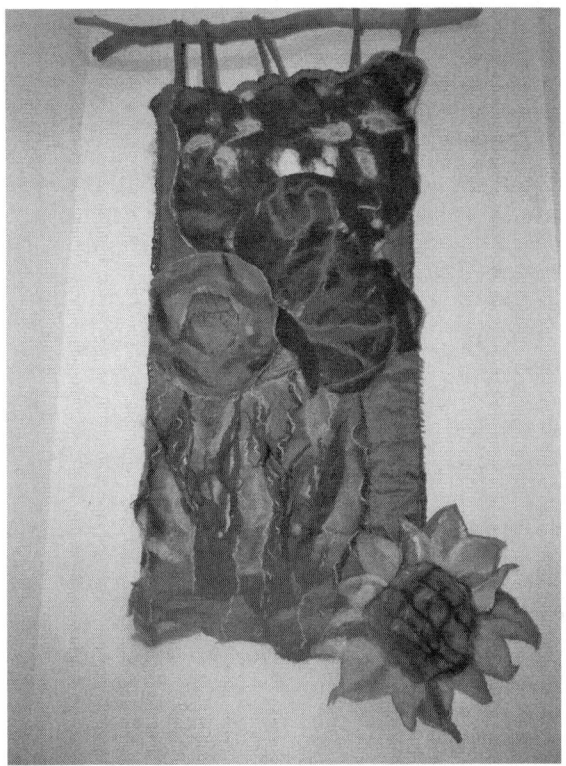

Figure 12.1 Journey: wall hanging incorporating felted imagery mounted on post-surgery "blanket" (Dokter, 2012)

support from hospital, Wallace Centre, colleagues, friends and family, recovery proved a long and arduous process. The period from diagnosis to completion of treatment took four to five months only. I returned to my academic work in November and clinical work in early spring.

I found that the treatment left me extremely tired, lacking in energy, and with a mountain to climb regarding trauma and body image processing. A drawing/writing journal of my treatment journey proved useful for processing, as my memory was patchy due to side effects of the medication. I had envisaged a slow improvement over time, supported by a phased return to work, but found it tended to be a process of up and down. I returned to a previous therapeutic relationship. Having been seriously ill as a child, some of that trauma needed to be reprocessed, as well as the renewed experience of vulnerability and mortality. The coaching to prepare for return to work was helpful in setting boundaries towards employers, as their expectation was similar to mine, but phased return in academia being for a much shorter time than in the NHS. Given my leadership roles in both organisations, I was interested to find that those types of responsibilities were the hardest to return to. I did not feel fit to lead others while I was still trying to refind myself.

Clinical supervision helped to support my return to work journey, as did the two OH departments. Fitness to work needed to be a process of negotiation between what I felt able to do, what others thought I should be able to do, external checks through supervision, and OH. A year after I received the diagnosis, I felt ready to see clients again. The latter was influenced by my energy levels but mostly my sense that I again could focus on the client with a good enough presence. On return to my "normal work load" I found that I needed to cut back on my demanding two jobs and was supported in early retirement on health grounds from the NHS. Work-life balance had come sharply into focus in my illness experience and self-care became a priority, rather than an add on.

Lisa's story

After diagnosis, I had five days before I began chemotherapy. I wanted to end my clinical work in the way I felt it needed, so it was as therapeutic as possible for each client. For one client, it was mutually difficult. Her story was complex, and she had begun, against all odds, to trust me. Telling her was hard and I was as professionally honest in that encounter as she required of me. Years later she has contacted me privately to thank me for our brief time together and how she remembers it as a good and healing encounter. Though therapist illness is shocking for clients and can trigger anger, feelings of rejection, etc., if it is handled therapeutically it can allow the client to meet a healthy adult part of themselves, as their care for another human being manifests.

As aggressive treatment progressed, I withdrew from work. My body, mind, and spirit endured a reduction to its deepest level of survival. The six cycles of chemotherapy, lumpectomy, and twenty sessions of radiotherapy saved my life, physically. In my being, I experienced realising my mortality. A moment I recall after coming down from a nap was my partner and children playing and laughing. Life would continue whatever my treatment outcome. This was simultaneously wonderful and devastating for me.

I was proud of working for the NHS. Walking down the street bald was a challenge to my sense of identity. I could not wear a wig; it moved under the playfulness of my children (one and five years) and hurt my head. The school playground is a levelling place of fitting in or feeling you do not. Once the shock passed on both sides I settled into my skin. I experienced a sense of OK-ness while walking around "naked" outside and inside. I experienced from our community a love and care that reminded me of our shared humanity.

I attended a Time to Retune break through Cancer Lifeline South West (CLSW). Three days with facilitators who served participants food, provided therapeutic groups, and taught relaxation and mindfulness. Our stories were shared and heard. The timing of the break, when treatment ended and I was facing a return to work, was pivotal.

I took voluntary redundancy after a phased return with an awareness that staying, in the context I returned to, would set my system up to be so distressed I would have no chance of remaining cancer free. I was too exhausted and fragile to be back at work. I had been off for a year after nine months of treatment. The expectation was clear – I needed to be functional as a therapist. My memory was sluggish, the fatigue immense, and there was no support at work.

A new supervisory relationship, therapy, and love enabled me to set up in private practice not knowing what the future held but having realised, while on chemotherapy, that I needed to return to working with children. Now I work hard to say "yes" to work where it feels right and say "no" to work that sets off my alarm bells. Who I share my work self with is as important as every other relationship. It works best when it feels right even if neither of us yet know why that is so.

The clients I saw before I was diagnosed, who waited to see me afterwards, are the people I found it hardest to work with. I had been right for them pre-diagnosis, but I was no longer the same person. I was irrevocably changed. I had gone back into therapy just before diagnosis. My therapist experienced bereavement within the time of our therapeutic relationship. I realise now, in the same way I feared for and felt for my own therapist in her loss, and was unsure how "we" would be on her return, was what was discordant for my own clients. How this is honoured, this profound shift in relationship, is key.

Tara's story

"But what do I tell the kids?" I could not think past that impossible question, while the medics who had just diagnosed me were trying to communicate treatment options. Aged fourteen I had watched my beloved Dad die from cancer at home. My siblings and I thought he had a particularly bad cold. Our parents had hoped that we would come to our own conclusions that Dad was dying as we saw him deteriorate. They had not reckoned on the power of the psyche to see what it wants to see rather than what is really happening. Now aged forty-seven, with twenty years of dramatherapy practice, and mother to three children, who were the same age as my siblings and I when Dad died, I knew I had to tell my kids the truth. The challenge was knowing what truth to tell? Having trained as an actor, I was adept at immersing myself into a role, using Stanislavski's "Method Acting." I convinced myself that my role was of someone who was going to survive cancer, and this is what I told myself and my three girls. I did not know that all my other roles in life were about to disappear.

I was pre-menopausal, but with my beautiful family complete, I need not fear infertility, and was accepting that my bikini days were over anyway. Thus, I stayed positive. It was not until much later that I re-engaged with

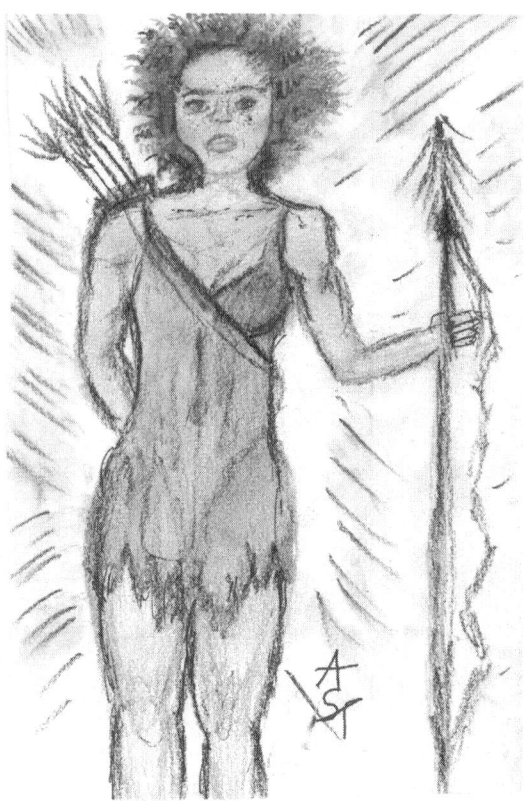

Figure 12.2 Single breasted Amazonian warrior, Autumn Skye Thornewood, 4 July 2016.

psychodynamic therapy. Before that, I was held completely by my family and by my closest friends (or, as we affectionately refer to ourselves collectively – "'burds' ... of a feather"). They cooked, cared, listened, offered their hair to make a wig, and ensured that one of them was with me at every medical appointment. Of most importance was the support of my three daughters who absolutely believed in my recovery.

I relinquished my identities of wife, mother, friend, daughter, sister, and dramatherapist, as these relationships had all taken an unrecognisable turn. Friends no longer confided their woes in me, my children no longer needed me to carry out domestic tasks, or comfort them emotionally, my husband no longer wanted to be near me for fear of "catching chemo," and all my therapy clients were simply getting on with their lives without me.

Rebuilding my identity is a "work in progress." The surgeons cut the cancer out of my body (after a gruelling five months of chemotherapy, followed by radiotherapy, and medication for ten years), but the cancer will never be completely gone. I can never get back to "normal." There is nothing linear, in my experience, about recovery. It is a roller coaster. What I am getting better at is living with it and nourishing every other aspect of who I am as much as possible.

Negotiating fitness to practice

Returning to work, after a potentially life-threatening illness, brings its own unique challenges. Diagnosis often comes as a sudden shock, guilt can be closely linked, as well as paralysing fear. (Re-)finding creativity post the trauma of life-threatening illness may assist the paralysis of fear to become transformed into new agency.

Art(s) therapists are used to adaptation – a theatrical term, as well as a necessary skill, when working psychodynamically, particularly with the body. Babette Rothschild (2000) refers to the body as an anchor, as gauge, and as break. Elsewhere in this chapter (see p. 000), we discuss the use of creativity in the healing process for the therapist – concurring with Anne Bannister's belief that creativity is the immune system of the psyche (Casson-Christie, 2015). Cancer treatments leave patients with a compromised immune system. The creative self, as a potential vessel for self-healing may completely disappear. Creativity requires significant risk taking, and this may simply not be possible. Physically disabling symptoms such as pain, limited mobility, high levels of adrenaline, toxic, destructive chemicals (such as chemotherapy) are placing the patient in survival mode. New ways of dealing with what happens during treatment, may need to be found.

One author's experience was that during chemotherapy she was immersed in sensation. Creativity was absent in the depths of treatment. This then shifted to emerging and finding creativity through healing body and mind – singing, walking, rescuing a Lurcher, running and psychotherapy ... Once they are accessible, expression, embodiment, and creativity may well form an integral part of recovery.

Dramatherapists using embodiment (Dokter, 2016a) may feel too subsumed in the body's destructiveness to be able to be creative. This loss of identity as a creative being can further debilitate the healing process as it throws up the question – "Who am I if I can no longer be true to my creative self and to my career? Will patients ever trust that I am safe again? How will I cope with suicidal patients, having fought so hard to preserve my own life? Is my life worth saving any more than anyone else's, when I see glimpses of how the world will continue to turn without me?"

Wadeson (2011) was an inspiration for the return to textile art as an alternative creative route, as seen in the wall hanging illustration (Dokter, 2012) – see Figure 12.1. Wadeson's coping mechanisms of journaling with drawings, writing, and poetry or passively listening to music, could be useful for others too, particularly when treatment involves isolation, which may be an unfortunate re-enactment of previous trauma.

With returning strength, it may be possible for dramatherapists to start re-engaging with their more familiar art form through embodiment, while learning to adapt to new (dis)abilities in relation to self, others, and their environment. Amerta movement (Bloom et al., 2014) was the inspiration for one author to join a creative project group, working together with others through movement to pursue individual creative projects (Dokter 2014, 2016b).

Cancer is not a one-off event. It is an ongoing process of trying to maintain balance between the euphoria of being a survivor and the ever-present reality check of being repeatedly exposed to near death, when signs and symptoms return. One of the biggest features of surviving cancer is the fear of recurrence (Horlick-Jones, 2011). How does a therapist continue to work, through each new "scare"? It is arguable that their capacity to connect with their creative selves may be an indication of whether they are starting to recover. Once able to risk take, by holding other's creativity, then it may be time to return to work.

Role of supervision

Supervision holds an intention to support therapist well-being and this is integral in our capacity to practice. Supervision cannot happen without a good working alliance. This requires formation of an attachment. Polyvagal theory proposes a bio-behavioural explanation for the relationship in therapy and how specific features of therapeutic presence trigger a neurophysiological state in both client and therapist within which both perceive and experience feelings of safety (Porges, 2001). Polyvagal theory proposes that a state of safety is mediated by neuroception, a neural process that may occur without awareness, which constantly evaluates risk and triggers adaptive physiological responses that respond to features of safety, danger, or life threat (Porges, 2001).

Similar features of relationship are fundamental to supervision. The supervisor of a therapist who has had a life-threatening illness may need to pay more attention to the state of the nervous system of the supervisee and be aware of the need to help the supervisee reflect upon when their fight/flight/freeze responses are too aroused. As therapists, our clients must be able to access a therapist with a settled nervous system in order that the necessary relationship can be built. "Recovery from trauma involves the restoration of executive functioning and, with it, self-confidence and the capacity for playfulness and creativity" (van der Kolk, 2014, p. 205).

Good supervision may not be enough to maintain therapist well-being. Supervision cannot address the build-up of stress or distress in the therapist or the intake of toxicity from client material or organisation that is contained within the body. A body-based supervision may go some way to making the same kind of shifts in energy required; exercise that increases the heart rate and releases endorphins is likely to be beneficial. Its arousal is similar to that of a distressed nervous system but releases toxicity.

Conclusion: work-life balance and therapist self-care

This chapter uses autoethnographic stories to study the experiences of three (drama)therapists with cancer and the impact on their practice and self-care.

Paying attention to therapist illness and its impact on client care is an important area of further arts therapies research – in particular, sickness incidence rates, rates of attrition from the profession, as well as types of illnesses developed in comparison with the general population. Additionally, self-care strategies to prevent and process health and illness experiences need further research.

References

Adams, M. (2014). *The myth of the untroubled therapist: Private life, professional practice*. London: Routledge.

Alker, G. (2015). A feminist rethinking of dramatherapy: The role of audience and aesthetics in cancer as change maker. *Dramatherapy Review*, 1(2), 187–199. Performance on https://www.youtube.com/watch?v=TjFne8FLpl.

Bloom, K., Galanter, M., & Reeves, S. (Eds.) (2014). *Embodied lives: Reflections on the influence of Suprapto Suryodarno and Amerta movement*. Axminster, UK: Triarchy Press.

Boehm, K., Cramer, H., Staroszynski, T., & Ostermann, T. (2014). Arts therapies for anxiety, depression and quality of life in breast cancer patients. *Evidence Based Complementary and Alternative Medicine*. (2014) 103297 Retrieved from www.ncbi.nlm.nih.gov/books/NBK200736.

Casson-Christie, J. (2015). Anne Bannister obituary. *The Guardian*, 6 April.

Dokter, D., Holloway, P., & Seebohm, H. (Eds.) (2011). *Destructiveness in dramatherapy*. London: Routledge.

Dokter, D. (2012). *Journey*. Retrieved from www.whitwellweaving.co.uk.

Dokter, D. (2014). *Finding home*. Westhay, Dorset, UK (September) Performance.

Dokter, D. (2016a). Embodiment in dramatherapy. In S. Jennings & C. Holmwood (Eds.) *International handbook of dramatherapy*. (pp. 115–125). London: Routledge.

Dokter, D. (2016b). *Come or go?* Charmouth, Dorset, UK (September2016). Performance. Retrieved from https://youtube.be/cCzq9CS_681.

Edwards, J. (2016). *When the therapist is ill*. Retrieved from www.contemporarypsychotherapy.org.volume-8-no1-summer-2016/when-the-therapist-is-ill/.

Freud, S. (1997). *Dora: An analysis of a case of hysteria*. New York: Touchstone Books (Original work published 1905).

Gergen, M. & Gergen, K. (2002). Ethnographic representation as relationship. In A. Bochner & C. Ellis (Eds.) *Ethnographically speaking: Autoethnography, literature and aesthetic* (pp. 11–33). Walnut Creek, CA: Altamira.

Goleman, D. (1995). *Emotional intelligence*. New York, Bantam Books.

Horlick-Jones, T. (2011). Understanding fear of cancer recurrence in terms of damage to 'everyday health competence'. *Sociology of Health and Illness*, 33(6) 884–898.

Johnson, W. B. & Barnett, J. E. (2012). When illness strikes you. What are your ethical obligations as a practitioner in the face of a life- threatening illness? *Monitor on Psychology*, 43(10), 50–55.

Jones, P. & Dokter, D. (Eds.) (2008). *Supervision in dramatherapy*. London: Routledge.

Kaufman, S. E. (2016). The effects of self-disclosure of a mental health condition on client perception of the therapist. Unpublished dissertation, Philadelphia College of osteopathic medicine. PCOM psychology dissertation Retrieved from www.digitalcommons.pcom.edu.

Levine, P. A. (2010). *In an unspoken voice: How the body releases trauma and restores goodness*. Berkeley, CA: North Atlantic Books.

Levy-Gigi, E., Bonanna, G. A., Shapiro, E. R., Richter-Levin, G., Keri, S., & Sheppes, G. (2015). Emotion regulatory flexibility sheds light on the elusive relationship between repeated traumatic exposure and PTSD symptoms. *Clinical Psychological Science*, (May 13, 2015), 1–12. doi:10.1177/2167702615577783.

Mullen-Williams, J. (2016). Translating the cultural subtext. In D. Dokter & M. Hills de Zarate (Eds.), *Intercultural arts therapies research* (pp. 172–190). London: Routledge.

North American Dramatherapy Association. Retrieved from www.nadta.org/membership/selfcare-for-therapists.html.

Pearlman, L. A. & McKay, L. (2008). *Understanding and addressing vicarious trauma*. Pasadena, CA: Headington Institute.

Porges, S. (2001). The polyvagal theory: Phylogenetic substrates of a social nervous system. *International Journal of Psychophysiology*, 42, (2001), 123–146.

Rothschild, B. (2000). *The body remembers*. London: W.W. Norton.

Scaer, R. (2014). *The body bears the burden*. London: Routledge.

Skovholt, T. M. & Trotter-Mathison, M. (2016). *The resilient practitioner* (3rd edn.). London: Routledge.

Stern, D. (1995). *The motherhood constellation. A unified view of parent-infant psychotherapy*. London: Routledge.

Stevens, A. (1994). *Jung*. Oxford: Oxford University Press.

van der Kolk, B. (2014). *The body keeps the score*. London: Penguin Random House.

van Maanen, J. (1988). *Tales of the field; on writing ethnography*. Chicago, IL: University of Chicago.

Wadeson, H. C. (2011). *Journaling cancer in words and images. Caught in the clutch of the crab*. Springfield, IL: Charles C. Thomas.

Wilton, A. (2001). The impact of illness on the therapist's self and the handling and use of this in therapy. *Reformulation* ACAT News Autumn2001(9). Retrieved from www.acat.me.uk/refomulation.php?issue-id=33&article-id=405.

Chapter 13

Movement observation in trauma-centred case supervision

Claire Schaub-Moore

Introduction

People who have experienced adverse life experiences (Felitti, 2002) usually need medical, psychotherapeutic, and/or social support because of the manifold acute and/or long-term consequences. It is well known that treatment models for traumatised people must be extensive (Herbert, 2006; Moore, 2007a, 2007b; Perry, 1995, 2001; Reddemann, 2001, 2004; van der Kolk et al., 1996, 2000). Working with people who have been through complex trauma is a constant challenge for professional helpers. In addition to their specialist skills and abilities, this work requires particular attention to how traumatic experiences can fundamentally influence, change, and shape people's lives. Regardless of the consequences, whether somatic, psychosomatic, psychological and/or social, the body is always actively involved and holds past and present experiences (Petzold et al., 2002), or, as van der Kolk (1994, title of his paper) put it: "The body keeps the score." Fragmentary aspects of previous and current (traumatic) experiences are conveyed and transmitted on a sensory, cognitive, emotional, and kinaesthetic level, regardless of what is said on a verbal level. This requires particular attention for the communication of the body, which can be seen in movements. The observable movements can be understood as unconscious movement preferences that a person uses to deal with experiences in the best possible way and are thus resources for further development.

An observation system that describes and interprets movement patterns with a theoretical framework, such as the Kestenberg Movement Profile (KMP) (Kestenberg Amighi et al., 2018), is valuable for working with people who have experienced traumatic incidents. In the following case study, the KMP is an essential part of case supervision. In order for this specific type of supervision to be helpful, the supervisees need to know the basics of the observation system without having to be movement analysts themselves. This expanded understanding of communication in professional situations can be particularly useful if case understanding and reflection is based on Reflected Casuistics (Adler, 1994; Geigges, 2002; Schaub, 2008; Uexküll & Wesiak, 1996); a psychodynamic technique that combines process- and goal-oriented diagnostics and a case study.

Supervision

The most commonly used method of reflection in clinical work is supervision. This approach can be applied with individuals, in groups or in teams, intended to support processes of change, stability, and development (Hausinger et al., 2007; Rappe-Giesecke, 2003; Schaub & Schwall, 1995). Supervision differs from consulting in reflexive reasoning and discursive communication about roles, assignments, and tasks in the job (Hausinger et al., ibid.).

Case supervision is based on the assumption that "nursing, medical, social or psychological work not only relies on its respective expertise, but also on how interactions with patients can benefit from the expertise" (Schaub 2008, p. 106; translated CSM). In order for this interaction to succeed, an understanding of communication processes, in particular the meaning of narratives, i.e. stories, between professional helpers and their patients/clients is crucial. Reflected Casuistics (Adler, 1994; Geigges, 2002; Schaub, 2008; Uexküll & Wesiak, 1996) supports the "dialogic principle" (Jakobs & Röh, 2005) between professional helpers and their patients/clients by combining process- and goal-oriented diagnostics and a case study. The interactions patients/clients have had with specialists are understood as "stories" that are looked at in their development over time. For the purpose of case supervision, Adler's approach has been modified to three perspectives of these "stories" (Schaub, 2008):

1   The (medical) story of the patient/client with the social and health care system and its interventions.
2   The (biographical) story of the person who has made contact with the social and health care system.
3   The story of the patient/client (system) with the institution carrying out the diagnostics and casuistry.

The aim of this chapter is not only to take up the dialogic principle of "stories" with an understanding for underlying messages in verbal language, but to expand it by an understanding of the meaning of non-verbal communication, particularly in the light of trauma. Subjectivity comes to the fore in dialogue. The inner perspective of subjectivity, however, can only partially be accessed linguistically. Movement observation may help to give it an expression.

Movement observation

The body is more than just an object, a "fixed, material entity subject to the empirical rules of biological science" (Csordas, 1994, p. 1). It is "the seat of subjectivity" (ibid., p. 9), "intercommunicative and active; and it is so through emotion" (Lyon & Barbalet, 1994, p. 48), indicating that bodies are social agents. The body thus potentially opens up space for reflection, thoughts, knowledge, and understanding of oneself in one's own history/story (Abrams,

1996). This story is marked by intra- and intersubjective experiences, in which culture, socialisation, education, interpersonal experiences, and religion form the body and its "language." "When we look at a body we are looking at the history of that body and the history of the difficulties in that body to body relationship" (Orbach & Carroll, 2006, p. 69). The knowledge of a self is always connected with the experience of having and being a body, on the basis of moving realities in the form of "substance, action, sensation, affect, and time" (Stern, 1985, p. 71).

Working with people who have experienced traumatic incidents, it is important to pay particular attention to the communication of the (therapist's and patient's) bodies and their "languages" through movement. The inclusion of body language as an expression of somatosensory memory (van der Kolk et al., 2000) considerably expands the medical, counselling, and therapeutic tools, as there is a chance of accessing both pre-verbal and non-verbal experiences. Furthermore, a sensory, kinaesthetic, and perceptual perception of the other can promote the working relationship in terms of interest, empathy, attunement, and an ability to work. The professional helper can use the principles of somatic countertransference by perceiving his or her own body, movements, feelings, fantasies, inner images, etc. in order to potentially establish a connection to the process of the patient/client and the intersubjective field (Orbach 1999; Carroll 2004).

Movement observation has a long and varied history as a discipline and is an essential therapeutic and diagnostic tool in dance movement psychotherapy (Berufsverband der TanztherapeutInnen Deutschland, BTD, 2006). Based on the theory of movement analysis by Rudolf von Laban (Laban, 1960), called Laban Movement Analysis (LMA), there is a series of complex movement observation systems today that analyse movements in inner and outer three-dimensional space (Bartenieff & Lewis, 1980; Cohen, 1993; Davis, 1988; Kestenberg Amighi et al., 2018; Lamb & Watson, 1979). The analysis of movement sequences can shed light on neurophysiological and psychological processes within a cultural/social context. These can be used for diagnostics as well as intervention and evaluated for the working alliance. Care must be taken to ensure that the movement observations are as neutral as possible. As Moore and Yamamoto (1988) explain, there is no one-to-one correlation between a movement and a meaning, or between a meaning and a movement, or between a meaning and an encoded movement. Movement observation is based on individual body experiences, on an understanding of the mover's personal history and cultural background, so that the interpretation of a movement can and must be individually different.

This chapter presents selected components of the relationship of *Body Effort Space Shape* (BESS) (Bartenieff & Lewis, 1980; Hackney, 1998) that the team had learned in an intensive two-days seminar (Moore, 2006, 2007b, 2008). The aim of imparting basic movement observation skills is to heighten awareness of non-verbal forms of communication so that this understanding can be used and evaluated adjunct to the "stories" of the patient/client.

Case study

Michael is introduced in the case supervision of the therapeutic and social work team of a residence for "young chronically mentally ill people." Michael is twenty-two years old and has been living there for eighteen months.

The procedure in supervision is based on the system of *Reflected Casuistics* (see p. 000). The team reports:

Story 1.

The following information can be taken from Michael's medical records:

- usual teething troubles
- up to age 9: frequently wets at night
- age 8: bruises in the rib area and on the back; cited cause: fell down the stairs from the first floor
- age 9: forearm fracture; cited cause: fell off ladder
- age 12: bloodshot right eye and swelling of the right side of the face; cited cause: fell off bicycle
- age 14–19: three admissions to psychiatric hospitals (see Story 2)

Story 2.

The following information is mainly derived from the team members' conversations with Michael, his mother, and the family doctor (Michael's father and his siblings took part in a family session at the residence).

Michael was born as the second son of a hotelier family in a city in Central Germany. His brother Daniel (+ 3 years) is a cook in his parents' hotel, his sister Margret (– 2 years) is training as a hotel manageress. The hotel was originally built by Michael's paternal grandfather after he had returned from Russian captivity in 1950. Like Michael and his family, Michael's father, born in 1953, grew up in the hotel with his younger brother and parents. Michael's mother, born in 1955, was working as a secretary in a tax office when she met her husband. After her marriage in 1981, she moved to the family hotel and has been working for the hotel ever since.

The successful hotel was run under the strictly patriarchal regime of Michael's grandfather until Michael's father took over as first-born in 1983. Despite their retirement, the grandparents still live in the hotel. Michael's father's brother had joined the navy at the age of nineteen and was thus "on a great journey." Michael never liked living in the hotel. At the age of six he had already said that he wanted a "real home." Nobody could understand him.

According to his mother, Michael was a rather shy, withdrawn child. In nursery, he preferred to play on his own, in primary school he had one friend who moved away at the beginning of the fourth grade. He did not develop any friendships worth mentioning in secondary school either. Michael had difficulties concentrating at school, so his performance was rather low. Nevertheless, he made the transition to secondary school.

Michael's passion was painting, and he could spend hours working with paper and pencils. At the age of twelve, he abruptly stopped painting after his father had praised him for a painting he had drawn at school. This, according to his father, "is when his illness broke out, he completely changed, turned aggressive, moody and disgusting." Michael increasingly retreated to his room, spent a lot of time at the computer, refused to eat with his family, and yelled at his mother and siblings when they wanted to get closer to him. His performance at school declined rapidly and his behaviour was marked by a complete withdrawal. The situation came to a head when Michael was fourteen years old. After repeated teasing by classmates, Michael beat a boy from his class and threatened him with a knife. The school alerted the parents and the youth welfare office who, jointly, decided to admit him to child and youth psychiatry.

When Michael was discharged after six weeks, the domestic situation worsened. Between the father and Michael fierce fights developed, which usually ended in scenes of violence and the disappearance of Michael for days. Michael only rarely contacted his counsellor who had been appointed by the district court. The school also increasingly reported him missing. Michael finally dropped out of school at the age of fifteen. Via the internet, Michael bought Valium, which he used in combination with alcohol. In a state of drunkenness, he was picked up by the police at the station at the age of sixteen and taken back to child and youth psychiatry.

After his second psychiatric stay, he lived in a psychosocial rehabilitation centre where he began training as a cook. After three months, Michael broke off and disappeared. At the age of seventeen, he was arrested again for excessive alcohol abuse. The doctors, therapists, social workers, Michael, and the family decided to make an attempt to bring Michael back home (to the hotel). Three times a week, he visited a day care centre where he was supposed to develop a day structure and career prospects. Parents, siblings, and paternal grandparents pressed for a "quick recovery," as, according to Michael, they found it "embarrassing, shaming for the business that I was ill." They were of the opinion that all he needed to do was "work then he will get better." At the age of nineteen, Michael tried to kill himself with pills. After eight weeks in the adult psychiatry, Michael moved back home and lived in his room until a place in the current residence became vacant.

Story 3.

Michael has been living in the residence for eighteen months.

Here, young adults live that have at least one psychiatric diagnosis. In a multidisciplinary team of therapists and social workers, the aim is to facilitate young people's transition to work and to a self-determined life. In addition to individual counselling, Michael regularly participates in group activities (cooking, shopping, sports, excursions) and has been enrolled in the evening school for six months where he wants to graduate from secondary school.

Although Michael regularly participates in the activities, the team worries about his contact difficulties, which usually show in complete withdrawal or in sudden aggressive verbal and physical attacks against roommates. In addition, team members report their own feelings of increasing resignation and anger. The counsellor, Mr Dell, puts it this way: "Somehow I'm turning in circles with him. Nothing seems to be getting to him. Sometimes I have the feeling that he lives on some other star – he looks right through me when I talk to him. I sometimes get so angry, I don't know what to do." The team members want to understand how they can get out of the "circle" and follow new paths of recovery with Michael.

Michael's first two "stories" are collected on flipchart paper. From the information, the team members filter out the terms that are important to them and write them next to the stories. The terms are: "he is merely functioning," "social isolation," "taciturn," "disgrace," "pressure," "violence," "suicide attempt," "discontinuities," "drugs over the internet." In order to discover possible connections between Michael's experiences and his forms of communication, Michael is next physically brought into space with the method of movement observation. Mr Dell is the first to embody Michael's movements. While Mr Dell walks around the room, the remaining team members observe and mirror him and write down their observations. Together, they try to find Michael in their movements. After about ten minutes of moving, the team members and I, their supervisor, sort their main observations in a BESS table. The physical sensations after moving are described as "grave/lethargic," "fear," "sad," and "void." The analysis of their movement observations indicates that Michael prefers to move with indulging, not fighting qualities. His breath is in the first position, i.e. in and above the collarbone. This might be an expression of (chronic) anxiety. This impression is reinforced by his downward gaze, which seems to avoid contact with the outside world. Michael's mostly spinal movements reflect the earliest phase of ego development, in which attention is usually directed inwards and experiences with others are made via sensory, proprioceptive, kinaesthetic impressions. Movements are mainly initiated by the head or the tailbone and enable the infant to move and develop gradually in relation to gravity (Hartley, 1995). Michael's increased tension in his arms and back might also be interpreted as an anxiety-induced posture of impending danger, unconsciously preparing him for fight, flight or freeze reactions.

In his use of *efforts* it seems that Michael has only few strong, direct, and quick/sudden impulses. According to Kestenberg Amighi et al. (2018) fighting qualities (strong, direct, quick/sudden) convey wishes and intentions very clearly. By contrast, Michael's more indulging qualities may indicate unresolved bodily residuals of powerlessness, indirectness, and deceleration or helplessness after traumatic experiences. It is interesting that Michael sometimes fights "eruptively," verbally and physically, so that it can be assumed that triggers bring out an innate readiness to fight. His ability to "fight" can be considered as a resource.

In *shape* Michael seems to unconsciously prefer closed forms on all three dimensions. According to Kestenberg Amighi et al. (ibid.), a persistent closure of the dimensions indicates states of anxiety and insecurity. The horizontal dimension stands above all for the development of self-perception, the vertical for the ability to assert oneself and to distinguish oneself from the environment, while the sagittal dimension represents the quality of interpersonal contact, especially with regard to the ability to act. In a "normal," healthy state, the body can grow and close relatively symmetrically on all dimensions, promoting physical and mental stability, and a sense of balance. In the event of trauma, however, the ability to open is severely restricted. In the event of severe trauma, the body forms such a narrow, fear-induced protective wall that communication between the inside and outside world can be completely broken off at any time. By closing and withdrawing the movements ("dissociative behaviour") the self can be protected, while the physical shell remains unprotected. This can be understood as a mechanism to protect the self from possible fragmentation.

With regard to spatial orientation, the team members state that Michael's kinesphere is predominantly small, and only "large" in his aggressive outbursts. The kinesphere is the invisible space around a person that serves as a boundary and personal protection. The smaller this space becomes, the lower is the defence; the larger it becomes, the more the self can be protected. Growing into space has an engaging quality, however, blurry, expansive boundaries can become attacking. This might also be understood as an (unconscious) active, albeit aggressive way of self-protection. Michael thus shows a great need for protection, and the inability to adequately differentiate himself in his relationship with others. The exclusive use of the low level in the room is also striking. The lower the spatial level, the closer the body approaches a defenceless, almost regressive posture, which is particularly emphasised by the head-tail connectivity (spinal movements in *body*).

In summary, Michael's unconscious movement preferences suggest that his issues are an urgent need for protection, fear, and insecurity and that he withdraws into his "own" intrapsychic world. These assumptions are supported on the one hand by the physical sensations of the team members after having "moved" Michael ("grave/lethargic," "fear," "sad," "void"). These physically evoked associations point to somatic countertransferences. On the other hand, the movement observations underline the assumption that Michael experienced early childhood traumas. In his "stories," domestic violence is explicitly mentioned. The remarkably frequent bone fractures during childhood, wetting up to the age of nine, social withdrawal tendencies, concentration difficulties, alcohol, and Valium abuse, and the suicide attempt at nineteen years coincide with symptoms described mainly as sequelae of domestic violence (Egle & Nickel, 1998; Moore, 2007b; Perry, 1995, 2001). A "healthy" reaction to volatile and unpredictable situations is to develop fear and seek protection. However, if the outer world does not provide an adequate shelter, the only way out is to retreat into the inner world or into an illusory world created by drugs, alcohol or other psychotropic substances. The psychologically and physically suffered pain can be reduced there, because on the one hand contacts with real existing, potentially threatening and violent people remain far outside, on the other hand the extero- and interoceptive senses are desensitized neurophysiologically. Michael's stories do not tell who may have supported him in his childhood; his mother seemed to have been too frightened and intimidated herself to protect Michael. His siblings adapted to the system "family in the hotel": this shows in their choice of career and their lack of understanding for their brother in family conversations. The grandfather is known for his "strict rule," and the grandmother shares the family incomprehension and shame about Michael's illness. It can be assumed that family violence was a taboo in the family, and talking about it would only have ended with further violence. Michael's destructive behaviour in adolescence probably showed healthy reactions to unhealthy living conditions. But since no one in the support system questioned Michael's experiences, he had to follow the path of inner retreat, which at times has auto-aggressive, self-damaging traits. After an unsuccessful attempt to end life; lethargy, fear, sadness, and void remain, as the team members felt it in their somatic countertransferences.

In the subsequent analysis of the working relationship between Mr Dell and Michael, the team discusses which possible feelings and states Michael unconsciously transfers to Mr Dell. Withdrawn far into his inner world, verbal language seeps away as a communicative medium with the outside world. Past and present experiences and impressions can hardly be communicated verbally. However, Michael's experiences remain in the body as an "outcome" (van der Kolk, 1994), and are expressed in his movements. Thus, his need for protection, the fear, his regressive withdrawal into a "safe" inner world can be read in his body language, as well as the cause as an underlying film. Sometimes, Michael, as well as Mr Dell, get angry ("fight"), a "normal" reaction to a subjectively experienced threat, e. g. violence; a reaction, however, that Michael was not able to activate in the traumatic situations of his childhood and youth.

All three "stories," the medical story, Michael's biographical story, and Michael's current story, with the psychosocial residence, result in a narrative that demands further developmental steps in case supervision. From the insight gained it becomes clear that Michael can hardly be reached in a verbal-oriented setting. Based on the assumption that Michael experienced early traumas through violence, it is important not only to enable him to experience empathic, safe and reliable relationships but also for him (and the team) to learn that his reactions were "healthy protective behaviours" in the traumatic situations, yet stand in his way today. He needs to be supported in developing an ego-mature communication. His unconscious desire for protection or for secure boundaries must come first so that Michael can develop more confidence in his affect control, his self-perception, and consequently in relating. Put into practice, this means that professional helpers have to pick up and understand Michael's non-verbal language in order to, at best, be able to talk to him non-verbally. For example, Michael's multi-faceted bodily withdrawal requires sensitive observation. His closing body shapes and his "speechlessness" can on the one hand awaken the need in others to caress him, to touch him, and thus protect and comfort him. For Michael, however, this might mean his spatial (and emotional) boundaries are being invaded, which, dependent on context and person, he can only defend with vehement and abrupt gestures and movements. On the other hand, his body shapes may also trigger feelings of help-lessness, despair, and resulting anger in others (countertransference). Michael thus remains stuck in interactive patterns that do not allow him any space for devel-opment. Professional helpers should therefore check their own physical and psy-chological reaction to Michael, with the option of opening the communication space for him and leaving it up to him to decide how to make contact and com-municate. The decisive factors for his further development are that Michael is seen, taken seriously, and accepted.

Four weeks later, in the next case supervision, the team reports that Michael seems "more relaxed," and he is even able to laugh now. When asked how this change occurred, they answer: "We did not urge him to be with others all the time. If he didn't want to come out of his room, we expressed our regrets, but let him be. If he didn't say a word while cooking, we still praised him, e.g. for his skills in cutting, and thanked him for the good food. But it wasn't just him we concentrated on, he was part of the group." Mr Dell adds: "I can also let go better, I don't wait for an answer when we have a conversation. I have more understanding for him. Yesterday, he told me a little bit about the past, and then it became clear that even as a small boy he was regularly beaten by his father, but above all by his grand-father. Terrible." The team now also seems more relaxed.

Discussion and outlook

The model of trauma-centred case supervision has some particular features:

- Based on Reflected Casuistics, it offers an extension of the perspectives from which the patient/client is discussed and experienced. The division into three "stories" (medical history, biographical history, and the con-stantly evolving history of the person with the institution that introduces the patient/client in case supervision) enables an unusual breadth and depth of reflection on care/treatment since not only the patient/client with his/her diagnoses, but above all the person with his/her experiences and personal culture, is in the foreground.
- In the case supervision described here, a fourth dimension of observation is added. Here the dialogic principle of "stories" is not only taken up with an understanding for messages in verbal language, but is extended by an understanding of the meaning of non-verbal communication.

- The movements of both the patient/client and the professional helper are included in the reflection process and described by means of movement observation. By sensitizing the sensory, kinaesthetic, and perceptual perception of the other, the complexity of the patient/client becomes noticeable and the latter appears not only as a resident of a social-psychiatric institution, but as a "unique person." At the same time, the focus on non-verbal language is also aimed at sharpening the perception of the professional helper with regard to countertransference phenomena.

Movement observation is not only a diagnostic tool but also part of a comprehensive "clinical finding." This goal- and process-oriented finding is generated from the "stories" of the patient/client and uses a new element, which is characterised by an in-depth observation and reflection process about the different communications and interactions in the intersubjective space.

All experiences are immediately physical: the body absorbs experiences, processes them, and shapes the person's somato-psycho-social self-awareness and sense of coherence. This is reflected in the quality and nature of a person's movements and becomes particularly visible after traumatic life events. Movement observation offers the chance to discover the healthy, strong, and protective potentials in people. Considering this, modern multi-modal trauma therapy and counselling should include body-related psychotherapy and counselling (e.g. trauma-centred dance and movement psychotherapy).

This chapter also argues that professional helpers should further their knowledge on the importance of the body in the therapeutic and counselling space. In addition to training in trauma therapy and counselling, a basic understanding of movement observation is invaluable.

References

Abrams, D. (1996). *The spell of the sensous: Perception and language in a more-than-human-world.* New York: Pantheon Books.

Adler, R. (1994). Die Verwirklichung des biopsychosozialen Modells. In T. v. Uexküll (Ed.) *Integrierte psychosomatische Medizin in Praxis und Klinik* (pp. 221–235). Stuttgart, Germany: Schattauer Verlag.

Bartenieff, I. & Lewis, D. (1980). *Body movement: Coping with the environment.* New York: Gordon and Breach Science Publishers.

Berufsverband der TanztherapeutInnenDeutschlandse.V. (BTD) (2006, March). Ziele der Tanztherapie. Retrieved from http://www.btd.de.

Carroll, R. (2004). Emotion and embodiment: A new relationship between neuroscience and psychotherapy. Unpubl. training manual. Retrieved from www.thinkbody.co.uk.

Cohen, B. B. (1993). *Sensing, feeling and action: The experiential anatomy of body-mind-centering.* Northampton, MA: Contact Editions.

Csordas, T. J. (1994). Introduction: the body as representation and being-in-the-world. In T. J. Csordas (Ed.). *Embodiment and experience: The existential ground of culture and self.* (pp. 1–24). Cambridge: Cambridge University Press.

Davis, M. (1988). Movement psychodiagnostic inventory: Guidelines for use and interpretation. Movement behavior assessment. Unpubl. manuscript. Laban Centre, Goldsmiths College, University of London. November.

Egle, U. & Nickel, R. (1998). Kindheitsbelastungsfaktoren bei somatoformen Störungen. *Zeitschrift Psychosomatische Medizin*, 44, 21–36.

Felitti, V. (2002). The relationship of adverse childhood experiences to adult health: Turning gold into lead. *Zeitschrift Psychosomatische Medizin*, 48(4), 359–369.

Geigges, W. (2002). Reflektierte Kasuistik als Instrument der Forschung und Lehre einer integrierten Medizin. In T. v. Uexküll, W. Geigges, & R. Plassmann (Eds.). *Integrierte Medizin*, (pp. 125–146). Stuttgart, Germany: Schattauer.

Hackney, P. (1998). *Making connections. Total body integration through Bartenieff fundamentals*. Amsterdam, Netherlands: OPA/Gordon and Breach Publ.

Hartley, L. (1995). *Wisdom of the body moving. An introduction to body-mind centering*. Berkeley, CA: North Atlantic Books.

Hausinger, B., Möller, M., & Fellermann, J. (2007). Supervision 2007: Entwurf zu einem. Grundsatzpapier. Unpubl. manuscript DGSv.

Herbert, C. (2006). Healing from complex trauma: An integrative 3-systems' approach. In J. Corrigall, H. Payne, & H. Wilkinson (Eds.). *About a body. Working with the embodied mind in psychotherapy* (pp. 139–161). Hove, UK: Routledge.

Jakobs, S. & Röh, D. (2005). Über die (Un)Möglichkeit einer Sozialen Diagnose. *Soziale Arbeit*, 54, 282–288.

Kestenberg Amighi, J., Loman, S., & Sossin, M. (2018). *The meaning of movement. Embodied developmental, clinical and cultural perspectives of the Kestenberg Movement Profile*. London: Routledge.

Laban, R. (1960). *The mastery of movement*. London: MacDonald & Paul Evans.

Lamb, W. & Watson, E. (1979). *Body code: The meaning in movement*. London: Routledge and Kegan.

Lewis, P. (1999). Outline for the Clinical Interpretation of the KMP with Adults. In J. Kestenberg Amighi, S. Loman, P. Lewis, & M. Sossin (Eds.). *The meaning of movement. Developmental and clinical perspectives of the Kestenberg Movement Profile* (pp. 309–341). Amsterdam: OPA/Gordon and Breach Publ.

Lyon, M. & Barbalet, J. (1994). Society's body: Emotion and the 'somatization' of social theory. In T. J. Csordas (ed.). *Embodiment and experience: The existential ground of culture and self* (pp. 48–66). Cambridge: Cambridge University Press.

Moore, C. (2006). Dance movement therapy in the light of trauma: Research findings of a multidisciplinary project. In S. C. Koch & I. Bräuninger (Eds.). *Advances in Dance/Movement Therapy. Theoretical Perspectives and Empirical Research* (pp. 104–115). Berlin, Germany: Logos Verlag.

Moore, C. (2007a). Neue Wege in der Traumatherapie für von Häuslicher Gewalt betroffene Frauen, Kinder & Jugendliche. *Psychologie in der Medizin*, 15(3), 22–30.

Moore, C. (2007b). Die tiefenpsychologisch fundierte Tanz- und Bewegungspsychotherapie als Behandlungsmethode für Frauen, Jugendliche und Kinder im Kontext häuslicher Gewalt (Doctoral thesis, CvO Universität Oldenburg, Germany, VI, 197 Bl. – Oldenburg). Retrieved from http://docserver.bis.uni-oldenburg.de/publikationen/dissertation/2007/mootie07/mootie07.html.

Moore, C. (2008). Bewegungsbeobachtung in psychosozialen Berufsfeldern. Unpubl. seminar script.

Moore, C. & Yamamoto, K. (1988). *Beyond words: Movement observation and analysis.* New York: Gordon and Breach Publishers.

Orbach, S. (1999). *The impossibility of sex.* Harmondsworth, UK: Penguin.

Orbach, S. & Carroll, R. (2006). Contemporary approaches to the body in psychotherapy. Two psychotherapists in dialogue. In J. Corrigall, H. Payne, & H. Wilkinson (Eds.). *About a body. Working with the embodied mind in psychotherapy* (pp. 63–82). London: Routledge.

Perry, B. (1995). Neurobiological sequelae of childhood trauma: Posttraumatic stress-disorders in children. In M. Murberg (Ed.). *Catecholamines in post-traumatic stress disorder: Emerging concepts* (pp. 233–255). Washington, DC: American Psychiatric Press.

Perry, B. (2001). The neurodevelopmental impact of violence in childhood. In D. Schetky & E. Benedek (Eds.). *Textbook of child and adolescent forensic psychiatry* (pp. 221–238). Washington, D.C.: American Psychiatric Press Inc.

Petzold, H. G., Wolf, H.-U., Landgrebe, B., & Josic, Z. (2002). *Das Trauma überwinden. Integrative Modelle der Traumatherapie.* Paderborn, Germany: Junfermann Verlag.

Rappe-Giesecke, K. (2003). *Supervision. Team und Gruppensupervision.* Berlin, Germany: Springer.

Reddemann, L. (2004). *Psychodynamisch Imaginative Traumatherapie. PITT – Das Manual.* Stuttgart, Germany: Pfeiffer bei Klett-Cotta.

Schaub, H.-A. (2008). *Klinische Sozialarbeit. Ausgewählte Theorien, Methoden und Arbeitsfelder in Praxis und Forschung.* Göttingen, Germany: Vandenhoek & Ruprecht unipress.

Schaub, H.-A. &. Schwall, H. (1995). Fallsupervision und Teamberatung in medizinischen und psychosozialen Institutionen. *Gruppenpsychotherapie und Gruppendynamik*, 31, 331–345.

Schrank, B. & Amering, M. (2007) 'Recovery' in der Psychiatrie. *Neuropsychiarie*, 21(1), 45–50.

Stern, D. (1985). *The interpersonal world of the infant.* New York: Basic Books.

Uexküll, v. T. & Wesiack, W. (1996). Wissenschaftstheorie: ein bio-psycho-soziales Modell. In T. v. Uexküll (Ed.). *Psychosomatische Medizin* (pp. 13–52). München, Germany: Urban & Schwarzenberg.

van der Kolk, B. (1994). The body keeps the score: Memory and the emerging psychobiology of post-traumatic stress. *Harvard Review of Psychiatry*, 1, 253–265.

van der Kolk, B., McFarlane, A., & Weisaeth, L. (1996). *Traumatic stress. The effects of overwhelming experience on mind, body, and society.* New York: The Guilford Press.

van der Kolk, B., McFarlane, A., & Weisaeth, L. (Eds.) (2000). *Traumatic stress. Grundlagen und Behandlungsansätze.* Paderborn, Germany: Junfermann.

Index

Entries in *italics* denote figures.

absorption (motoric field) 60, 65
abuse, and trauma 1; *see also* domestic
abuse; sexual abuse; violence, family
accidents, trauma due to 1
activation (motoric field) 60
adaptation, in arts therapy 151
alcohol 37, 84, 100–1, 159, 161–2
amygdala 92, 145
anxiety: and armed conflict 52–3;
existential 8; in movement observation
160–1; in psychodrama 71, 73; of
therapists 34, 38
art: interrelatedness of 125; by therapists
147, 150, 151–2
arts therapies 2–4, 43, 103, 114, 153;
see also integrative arts psychotherapy
atemporality 47, 51, 53
attachment, repairing 93–4
attachment trauma 8, 58–9, 81, 83, 92
attentional recovery 134
attunement: child-carer 46–7, 59, 62,
77; non-verbal 83; therapeutic 3,
40–1, 70
autoethnography 146
autonomic nervous system 39, 62,
64, 133
autonomy 10–11, 95

baby-carer exchanges 46–7, 58–9, 76
Bannister, Anne 151
Bausch, Pina 12
belonging 11
Benjamin, Jessica 11
BESS (Body Effort Space Shape) 157, 160
bodily based approach *see* somatic
therapeutic approach

body: as container 136; language of 156–7,
162; negative self-images of 95; trauma's impact on the 19–20, 57–8, 92, 144
body actions 84
body experience: capacity to integrate
84–5, 87; music as 46
body image processing 147
body ownership 82, 84
body-related psychotherapy 2–3, 61–5, 164
boundaries: lack of 96; stabilising 98
Bourgeois, Louise 119
BPD (borderline personality disorder) 3,
88; biosocial model of 81–2; and resilience 82; and trauma 59, 80–1
Brandes, Vera 33
the breach 105
breast cancer 145–6
breathing: in baby-carer relationship 59;
in DMP 85, 88; traumatic patterns of
57, 64, 124
Broca's area 37, 124
Bucci, Wilma 128

canalisation (motoric field) 60
cancer, therapists living with 144–53
Casablanca 45, 48
CCPT (child-centred play therapy) 3,
34–41
chemotherapy 148–51
child-centred play therapy *see* CCPT
child-centred therapy 34
children, traumatised 26–7, 38–9
choreographic process 93, 100
closed dimensions 161
CLSW (Cancer Lifeline South West) 148
collective trauma 7, 23–4
combat veterans 3, 107–13
commonality 83

9781138479210